Healthcare Facility Planning

Thinking Strategically

Carrie Rich

Healthcare Facility Planning

Thinking Strategically

Cynthia Hayward

ACHE Management Series
Health Administration Press
Chicago, IL

Your board, staff, or clients may also benefit from this book's insight. For more information on quantity discounts, contact the Health Administration Press Marketing Manager at (312) 424-9470.

This publication is intended to provide accurate and authoritative information in regard to the subject matter covered. It is sold, or otherwise provided, with the understanding that the publisher is not engaged in rendering professional services. If professional advice or other expert assistance is required, the services of a competent professional should be sought.

The statements and opinions contained in this book are strictly those of the authors and do not represent the official positions of the American College of Healthcare Executives or of the Foundation of the American College of Healthcare Executives.

10 09 08 07 06   5 4 3 2 1

Library of Congress Cataloging-in-Publication Data

Hayward, Cynthia
   Healthcare facility planning : thinking strategically / Cynthia Hayward.
   p. cm.
   Includes bibliographical references.
   ISBN 1-56793-247-9 (alk. paper)
   1. Health facilities—Design and construction. 2. Health facilities—Planning. 1. Title.

RA967.H39 2005
725'.5–dc22

2005051348

The paper used in this publication meets the minimum requirements of American National Standard for Information Sciences—Permanence of Paper for Printed Library Materials, ANSI Z39.48-1984. ∞ ™

Acquisition manager: Janet Davis; Project manager: Jane Calayag Williams; Cover designer: Betsy Perez

Health Administration Press
A division of the Foundation of the
   American College of Healthcare Executives
1 North Franklin Street, Suite 1700
Chicago, IL 60606-3424
(312) 424-2800

Brief Contents

Detailed Contents

Preface

"We haven't the money, so we've got to think."

—Lord Rutherford
1871–1937

WHEN IT COMES to facility planning trends and capital investment, I have a tendency to divide healthcare organizations into the "haves" and the "have nots." The haves are those well-endowed and profitable healthcare organizations that maintain a continuous cycle of renewing and regenerating their facilities. Their investments in new or renovated facilities are generally well thought out and frequently visionary, even though their capital dollars are occasionally spent on oversized or inappropriate projects. The chief executive officers (CEOs) and board members of these organizations often take great pride in playing the role of the "master builder" and point to new "bricks and mortar" as part of their legacy. Whether their success is the result of the genius of their strategies or is simply a function of being in the right place (market) at the right time, their customers—patients, employees, and physicians—ultimately derive substantial benefit from their expenditures.

On the other hand are the have nots. Many healthcare organizations are still in survival mode and have not been able to focus on investing strategically in the future. According to the American Hospital Association (2005), 60 percent of U.S. hospitals lose money providing patient care and one-third lose money overall. Such financial pressures make it difficult for these healthcare organizations to make critical investments in their facilities. These organizations struggle to break even in more demographically challenged markets, experience limited negotiating leverage with payers, and find that sufficient capital is hard to obtain at their current levels of performance and cash flow. They must continue to squeeze the last bit of life out of their aging facilities with inadequate capital for retooling and renewal. Their dedicated staff use their expertise and empathy to create a "healing environment." While curtailing capital spending can be a useful short-term strategy to preserve liquidity, it leads to long-term problems that are very hard to solve, including the rising age of the physical plant.

This observation is substantiated by the widening credit gap between strong and weak healthcare providers. In 2004, there were 35 bond-rating upgrades for health systems and acute care hospitals, compared to 45 downgrades. Standard & Poor's (2005) anticipates that many providers will see a continuation of solid operating performance and growth in liquidity, while others will still have difficulty and experience further deterioration in credit quality.

Regardless of the financial situation, perspective, and culture of healthcare organizations, very few of them have capital to spend on inappropriate or unnecessary renovation or construction projects. Moreover, planning a major renovation project, or a new healthcare facility, is a rare opportunity for an organization to rethink its current patient care delivery model, operational systems and processes, and use of technology. A major investment of dollars in healthcare facilities should result in enhanced customer service, improved operational efficiency, potential new revenue, and increased flexibility, in addition to aesthetically pleasing, better-engineered, and code-compliant buildings that are the products of architects and engineers. At the same time, new or renovated facilities being planned today must be responsive to the needs of patients, caregivers, and payers in the twenty-first century and beyond.

The focus of this book is on predesign planning—a stage of the healthcare facility planning, design, and construction process that is frequently overlooked as organizations eagerly jump from strategic (market) planning into the more glamorous phase of design, which is typically led by an enthusiastic architect. During predesign planning, the healthcare executive has the greatest opportunity to express his or her vision for the organization, influence the nature of the process (top-down or bottom-up approach), and provide input relative to the future services to be provided—their size, their location, and their financial structure. Decisions made during predesign planning also have the most impact on long-term operational costs, compared to the initial cost of the bricks and mortar. Considering that buildings constructed today may be used for a half-century or more, the time spent on predesign planning provides a disproportionately large return on investment.

This book is intended as a practical guide and is based on my 25 years experience as a predesign planning consultant, assisting health-care executives and boards in optimizing their facility investments and providing future flexibility. I hope that this book will help you to under-stand the importance of the predesign planning process and to tailor the process to the unique needs of your organization. By deploying an integrated facility planning process, understanding the trends that affect space allocation and configuration, and planning flexible facilities, you can move confidently from planning to implementation.

REFERENCES

American Hospital Association. 2005. *The Fragile State of Hospital Finances.* [Online information; retrieved 7/21/05.] http://www.ahapolicyforum.org/ahapolicyforum/whatsnew/index.html.

Standard & Poor's RatingsDirect. 2005. *U.S. Not-for-Profit Health Care 2005 Outlook: The Calm Before the Storm.* [Online information; retrieved 5/9/05.] http://www.ratingsdirect.com.

Acknowledgments

I HAVE LEARNED a tremendous amount about facility planning from my clients over the years. I am particularly grateful to my clients who generously allowed me to include portions of their capital investment strategies and facility planning initiatives in this book, including the leadership team at the Lee Memorial Health System in Fort Myers, Florida, particularly David Kistel, vice president of facilities and support services. This dedicated and visionary group of executives not only understands the importance of developing a systemwide long-range capital investment strategy but also has been able to successfully implement its strategy over a multiyear period. I would also like to thank Rick Mace and Richard Haas at the Kettering Medical Center Network in Dayton, Ohio, for allowing me to include their innovative plan for reconfiguration of existing "hospital" space to enhance customer service and outpatient convenience, facilitate the efficient use of resources, and provide long-range physical and operational flexibility.

Other clients who contributed, knowingly or unknowingly, to this book include the leadership team at Mount Sinai Medical Center and Miami Heart Institute in Miami Beach, Florida, particularly Amy Perry, chief operating officer, and Steven Sonenreich, president and chief executive officer. I would also like to thank Gail Costa, vice president for planning at the Care New England Health System in Providence, Rhode Island; Christopher Male, senior vice president at Parrish Medical Center in Titusville, Florida; and the leadership teams at Hackensack University Medical Center in Hackensack, New Jersey, and Northwestern Memorial Hospital and the Northwestern Memorial Faculty Foundation in Chicago.

Audrey Kaufman and Janet Davis at Health Administration Press enthusiastically shared my vision for this book, and no author could ask for better assistance.

Needless to say, no work like this can be completed without the support of family and friends. My husband, Peter, provided unwavering support, common sense, and humor throughout this process. I am also very grateful to my deceased father, James R. Hayward, who taught me the art of critical thinking and to not be afraid to challenge commonly held perceptions and assumptions.

CHAPTER ONE

Rethinking the Facility Planning Process

W ITH ALL THE dramatic changes in the healthcare industry in the past 50 years—sometimes involving 180-degree shifts in popular trends and incentives—it is not surprising that many healthcare facilities become functionally obsolete even when their physical lives are not yet exhausted. Because of the lengthy facility planning process, new or renovated facilities that are just starting operations today may have been planned five or even ten years ago; yet these facilities are expected to endure for half a century or more. The question is, how can we ensure that the facility planning carried out this year or the next will produce facilities that are responsive to the needs of patients, caregivers, and payers in the year 2010, 2020, and beyond?

THE TRADITIONAL FACILITY PLANNING PROCESS IS PART OF THE PROBLEM

Historically, facility planning was project driven and often based on the wish lists of department managers, recruiting promises to physicians, and directives from donors. Large amounts of space and new facilities were part of the "arms race" among physicians and between department managers, both internally and with competing organizations. Appreciation (or recognition in budgeting) of space as an expensive resource was limited. Capital expenditures for facilities were not always coordinated with the institution's strategic planning initiatives, operations-redesign efforts, and planned information technology (IT) investments. A "build it and they will come" approach sometimes sufficed in lieu of a sound business plan. The impact of facility investments on long-term operational costs was frequently overlooked. Design and construction professionals tended to focus on the construction or renovation "project" and had little incentive to look for creative ways to avoid building. Moreover, facility projects were seldom viewed as part of an overall capital investment strategy for the organization (Hayward 2004).

Hospitals that follow this traditional facility master planning process find that their boards deny many projects, not only because of lack of capital but also because the project's impact on operational costs was not identified. Projects are often postponed indefinitely or downsized, and morale suffers when unmet expectations are communicated back to disillusioned physicians and department managers. This process often reminds me of the circus clown who opens a tin can out of which things pop out only to have to stuff the contents back into the can soon after.

When faced with a facility planning project that has taken on a life of its own, healthcare leaders must sometimes make the difficult and unpopular decision to stop or slow the planning or design process to reevaluate the need for the project and the effectiveness of the planned solution. At one critical point in the facility planning and design process, everyone involved focuses only on whether the project is "on time" and "on budget" and forgets about whether it is "on target" and is the right solution to the specific problem (Hayward 1995).

Today, successful healthcare organizations are deploying a more comprehensive, integrated, and data-driven facility planning process. This process begins with the strategic direction for the organization and integrates facility planning with market demand and service line planning, operations improvement initiatives, and anticipated investments in new technology. Major facility renovation and reconfiguration projects should not be planned without a foundation of data and analyses, including business plans for key clinical service lines, a review of institutionwide operations-improvement opportunities, an understanding of the project's impact on operational costs, and coordination with the organization's IT strategic plan.

THE NEW PLANNING ENVIRONMENT

The U.S. healthcare industry is in a crisis, dealing with fluctuating demand and utilization, capacity constraints, staffing shortages, intense media attention to patient safety, increased focus on information management, technology adoption and deployment challenges, rapidly rising costs, aging facilities, limited access to capital, and the new consumerism among healthcare users. All of these current issues affect the way facilities are used, planned, financed, and built.

Fluctuating Demand and Utilization

In a sharp contrast to the trends in the 1990s, today's environment is marked by increased demand for inpatient care, causing many healthcare organizations to focus attention back to their inpatient facilities, after a decade of concentrating almost exclusively on outpatient growth. While the upward trend in outpatient volumes has not subsided, the downward trend in inpatient volumes began modulating in the mid-1990s. Since the past decade, many factors have been at work to push down the inpatient component of hospital volume, such as payer pressures to limit admissions and reduce lengths of stay; new drugs and advances in technology, which allow patients to be effectively treated in an outpatient setting; and the creation of alternative settings to expensive inpatient care, including home health and skilled nursing facilities (AHA and Lewin Group 2004).

However, competing factors are contributing to an increase in inpatient utilization, including a growing and aging population, improved diagnostic techniques that find more people with illnesses, and new procedures that add to the range of treatment options. More recently, the loosening of managed care restrictions (allowing more patients to be treated in hospitals) and reductions in Medicare reimbursement for skilled nursing facilities and home health care have fueled inpatient utilization in acute care hospitals. In 1999, inpatient days in community hospitals increased slightly after two decades of decline, and they have increased steadily since then (AHA and Lewin Group 2004). This change comes at a time when many hospitals have substantially reduced the resources allocated for inpatient care, are experiencing limited access to capital for facility renovation and expansion, and are facing widespread staffing shortages.

Emergency departments (EDs) are undergoing similar fluctuations in demand. For example, ED visits increased in the early 1990s in proportion to the overall growth in the U.S. population while ED visits declined in the mid-1990s, as the U.S. population continued to rise. By the late 1990s, ED visits had increased almost three times the rate of population increase presenting a significant challenge for facility planners (AHA and Lewin Group 2004).

Capacity Constraints
Fewer hospitals exist today than in 1980 because of hospital closures and consolidations, which were in response to declining inpatient utilization and pressures to increase efficiency (AHA and Lewin Group 2004). Now that demand for hospital services is rising, many healthcare organizations are experiencing moderate-to-severe capacity constraints. From my experience, bottlenecks in EDs, intensive care units, and surgery suites are becoming increasingly common. This trend is particularly evident in the ED, because it not only serves as a key access point for emergency, episodic care but also functions as a safety net for America's 45 million uninsured people who have nowhere else to go for any level of medical care (DeNavas-Walt, Proctor, and Mills 2004). According to an American Hospital Association (AHA 2002) survey of hospital leaders, 24 percent of hospitals reported that their EDs are "at capacity," and another 24 percent reported that they are "over capacity."

Staffing Shortages
Even with adequate facility capacity, many healthcare organizations cannot find the staff to handle increased workload volumes. The National Center for Health Workforce Analysis (2002) estimated a shortage of almost 150,000 registered nurses (RNs) by 2005, increasing to 800,000 by 2020 as a result of the aging and retirement of nurses; enrollment in health education programs has been declining as well. Legislatively mandated nurse-to-patient ratios, such as in the state of California, and a wave of unionization activity across the country are taking the nursing crisis to a new level. Many other categories of healthcare workers are also in short supply, including pharmacists and imaging technologists. Healthcare organizations often expand their facilities only to find that they cannot staff them (AHA 2002).

Intense Media Attention to Patient Safety
In December 1999, the Institute of Medicine (IOM), an arm of the

National Academy of Sciences, published, *To Err Is Human*, a report that estimates that some 98,000 deaths and more than a million injuries occur each year as a result of medical errors (Kohn, Corrigan, and Donaldson 2000). Following the publication of this IOM report, additional studies at major medical universities and healthcare organizations around the world have advanced our understanding of how these medical errors occur. The focus on patient safety has led healthcare organizations to redesign work processes and to implement new technology, such as barcoding, and to evaluate the impact of facility design, such as a standardized layout for inpatient rooms and treatment spaces, on hospital error reduction.

Increased Focus on Information Management

In the effort to improve operational performance in the healthcare industry, the most common challenge is not planning space or even staffing but managing critical information. Completing paperwork requires at least 30 minutes, and often as much as 1 hour, for every hour of patient care provided (AHA 2002; PricewaterhouseCoopers 2001). It also makes the job of the healthcare provider less rewarding. Although, in my experience, recent technology advances and increased investment in healthcare IT help organizations to manage patient information, achieving a positive return on IT investments remains a current issue in the healthcare industry. The redesign of operational processes and the space in which they are performed is not always addressed concurrently with technology deployment. The provision of adequate staff education and training, as well as consideration of cultural and human factors, is also often lacking.

Technology Adoption and Deployment Challenges

New and innovative technologies are being developed on a daily basis to improve the patient's quality of life and longevity, to increase staff productivity, and purportedly to reduce ongoing operational costs. Many technologies that are already widely used in other industries are being adapted for the healthcare industry. Some new technologies that are having a significant effect on the utilization of staff, equipment, and space include the following:

- *Communication technologies*: integrated voice, data, and image fiber-optic telecommunication systems; satellite teleconferencing; intelligent networks; facsimiles; radio modems; and cellular phones

- *Biotechnology*: monoclonal antibodies, DNA probes, psycho-neuroimmunology, growth factors, gene splicing, bioregeneration of body parts, and new drug delivery systems

- *Bionics*: nerve chips and bioelectrical interfaces, healing electrical currents, magnetic fields, biochips, and inorganic body replacement parts

- *Miniaturized technologies*: nanotechnology, molecule-sized motors and machines that permit interbody diagnosis and repair, and portable/mobile diagnostic and treatment devices

- *Conscious technologies*: networked, computerized knowledge-based systems and devices dominated by artificial intelligence; self-learning computers; holographic three-dimensional animated computer-aided design; and virtual reality computer systems

- *Computerized, automated production technologies*: intelligent machine workstations and computerized flexible integrated manufacturing (CFIM) systems

- *Revolution in the capabilities of materials*: room-temperature superconductors, new alloys, new ceramic replacements for metals, carbon fiber technologies, and fiber optics

- *New energy systems*: high-efficiency batteries and room-temperature superconductor magnets

These new technologies are beginning to influence medical practice patterns and to create new possibilities for patient diagnosis and treatment. Often, less space is needed in large, centralized departments as equipment is miniaturized, made more mobile, and decentralized to the point of care. The sharing of data electronically via secure networks also eliminates the need for physical proximity of departments and functions, which was deemed necessary in the past. Less space is also needed for staff who may telecommute and for on-site hard-copy record storage. Because of the rate of change in healthcare technologies, healthcare providers and facility planners must monitor and assess new technologies (Hayward 2004).

Rapidly Rising Costs

Healthcare organizations are facing rapidly increasing costs, particularly those related to labor, professional liability coverage, drugs and biologics, new regulations, and disaster preparedness. In addition to complying with unfunded federal mandates, such as the Health Insurance Portability and Accountability Act (HIPAA) that took effect in 2003 and that set a national standard for medical privacy and transmission of electronic data, hospitals must also be on the front line in the event of disasters and must spend significant dollars to improve their capacity to respond to biological, chemical, and nuclear attacks (AHA 2002).

Aging Facilities

Healthcare organizations, like most businesses, need to continually maintain and update their physical plants to meet changing demand and to accommodate new technology. However, the investment required for healthcare facilities today is staggering because of the high costs of technology deployment; regulatory compliance; and physical plant upgrades, which may have been deferred for decades. From 1990 to 2003, the median average age of hospital physical plants in the United States increased from 7.9 years to 9.8 years (Ingenix and HFMA 2002).

Limited Access to Capital

While healthcare organizations are experiencing skyrocketing costs, their access to capital is becoming increasingly difficult. Hospital balance sheets remain weak, and sustained profitability is needed before access to capital can return to 1997 levels.[1] Wall Street's slump is also having a major impact on the healthcare economy: the market value of hospital investment portfolios dropped by 30 percent to 40 percent from 2000 to 2002 (Jaklevic 2002). Even with the recent upturn in the stock market, investment income will most likely not help many healthcare organizations offset operating losses.

The New Consumerism

A new consumer-driven market is emerging at the same time that the healthcare industry is experiencing rising costs, limited access to capital, and an expanding population of the uninsured. Consumers are paying more of their health plan and medical bill costs as employers and health plans shift more costs to enrollees. In 2004, enrollment in preferred provider organizations (PPOs), which provide a broader network and increased access to providers, outnumbered enrollment in health maintenance organizations (HMOs)—109 million compared to 68.8 million (InterStudy Publications 2004).

The aging baby boomers are also fueling the new consumerism. Better-educated and empowered by the Internet, they not only have the analytical ability to review research and form opinions about treatment options but also seek out what they perceive as the most healing environment and spend substantial discretionary income on their healthcare needs (Herzlinger 2002).

UNDERSTANDING THE NEW VOCABULARY

Rethinking the facility planning process also requires the use of new terminology, as shown in Figure 1.1. Strategic (market) planning has become more focused on financial viability, and so should healthcare organizations rely on a capital investment strategy rather than the traditional facility master plan to balance the trade-offs between investments in new "bricks and mortar," medical equipment and IT, ventures with physicians, and so on. Space planning, particularly for a major clinical service line, cannot be accomplished without a business plan that describes the market dynamics; expected workload volumes (revenue); and ongoing operational costs, particularly for staffing. Planned operational processes and new technologies to be deployed must also be defined and documented before space requirements can be determined. I prefer to use the term operational and space programming to describe the traditional space planning process, replacing the more recent term of functional and space programming, to emphasize the rigor that is required in rethinking operational processes before planning the physical space.

Even the traditional equipment planning process has changed. Most major equipment items use digital technology that must be planned in conjunction with the organization's overall information management strategy and technology planning. With electronic information exchange replacing the traditional flow of paper (and people), physical proximities that were once considered necessary are being reevaluated and new settings for delivering patient care are being con-

FIGURE 1.1   UNDERSTANDING THE NEW FACILITY PLANNING VOCABULARY

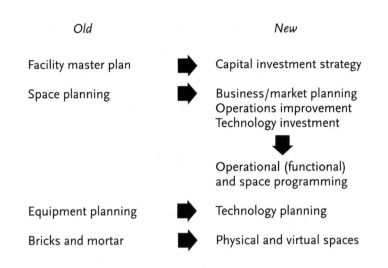

Old		New
Facility master plan	➡	Capital investment strategy
Space planning	➡	Business/market planning Operations improvement Technology investment ⬇ Operational (functional) and space programming
Equipment planning	➡	Technology planning
Bricks and mortar	➡	Physical and virtual spaces

sidered. As a result, the traditional bricks-and-mortar concept is being replaced by a combination of physical and virtual spaces.

THE CHALLENGE OF PREDESIGN PLANNING

The planning and delivery of a major capital project can be divided into six stages, as shown in Figure 1.2. The first stage of predesign planning—the focus of this book—includes general concepts and ideas in the form of words, numbers, and conceptual diagrams. Preliminary space estimates are used to develop a facility master plan and to generate project cost estimates early. Once specific projects are identified and approved, the detailed operational and space programming begins; when this is completed, the design architect can start the schematic design stage. Each subsequent phase brings more knowledge and detail about the project and has its own cast of players. Nearing the final phases, the concepts and ideas are translated into tangible architectural floor plans, drawings of construction details, and the eventual reality of the three-dimensional building (Waite 2005).

Predesign planning can be defined as the process of determining the following (Hayward 2004):

FIGURE 1.2 SIX STAGES OF A CAPITAL PROJECT

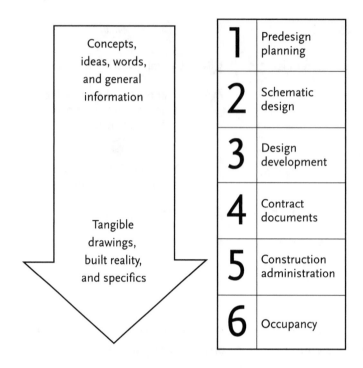

Source: Reprinted with permission from Waite, P. S. 2005. *The Non-Architect's Guide to Major Capital Projects: Planning, Designing, and Delivering New Buildings*. Ann Arbor, MI: Society for College and University Planning.

- *Right services* consistent with the organization's strategic initiatives, market dynamics, and business plan, at the

- *Right size* based on projected demand, staffing, equipment, technology, and desired amenities, in the

- *Right location* based on access, operational efficiency, and building suitability, with the

- *Right financial structure*—for example, owning, leasing, or partnering.

Predesign planning is the stage where the healthcare executive has the most influence on the potential success of the final project. His or her opportunity for input decreases as each subsequent stage passes. The opportunity to reduce both the initial capital cost and the ongoing operational costs is also greatest during the predesign planning stage, as shown in Figure 1.3. With the prospect of a new building project, healthcare executives tend to short-circuit or bypass the predesign stage to rush into the more tangible aspect of design. This is a big mistake. A premature focus on a construction or renovation project, without the rigor of the predesign planning process and the context of an overall capital investment strategy for the organization, often results in inappropriate and overbuilt facilities and increased operational costs that may not be justified by revenue growth. This is also a mistake, given that you, your organization, and your predecessors will have to live with the results of your project for a half-century or more. Predesign planning is critical from a short-term perspective: it is needed to design and construct a building that meets the needs of the first set of occupants. Predesign planning is also critical to the building's long-range functional life and its adaptability to accommodate future changes in medical practice, technology, and patient care.

According to Waite (2005), predesign planning is the part of the process where nonarchitects are the most involved. He cautions against engaging a design consultant prematurely: "Architects and engineers are energetic, creative problem solvers who are really good at what they do. But until your institution has worked through some of the steps of pre-design, you don't know if your problem is really a design problem or some other kind of problem. There are architects who tend to see all problems as design problems, even when they are actually management or organizational problems. A management or organization problem can often be solved internally by a policy decision rather than a design, thus saving a lot of time and money."

THE INTEGRATED PREDESIGN PLANNING PROCESS

Figure 1.4 illustrates the integrated predesign planning process that can be used by healthcare organizations to reconfigure existing facilities and to plan new facilities. The predesign planning activities shown in the diagram are separated into two:

1. *Capital investment strategy development and approval*: this includes five major activities (replacing the traditional facility master planning process).

FIGURE 1.3 IMPACT OF PREDESIGN PLANNING ON POTENTIAL CAPITAL/OPERATIONAL COSTS

Potential Capital/Operational Cost Savings

$

Predesign planning

Schematic design

Design development

Contract documents

Construction administration

Occupancy

Stages Over Time

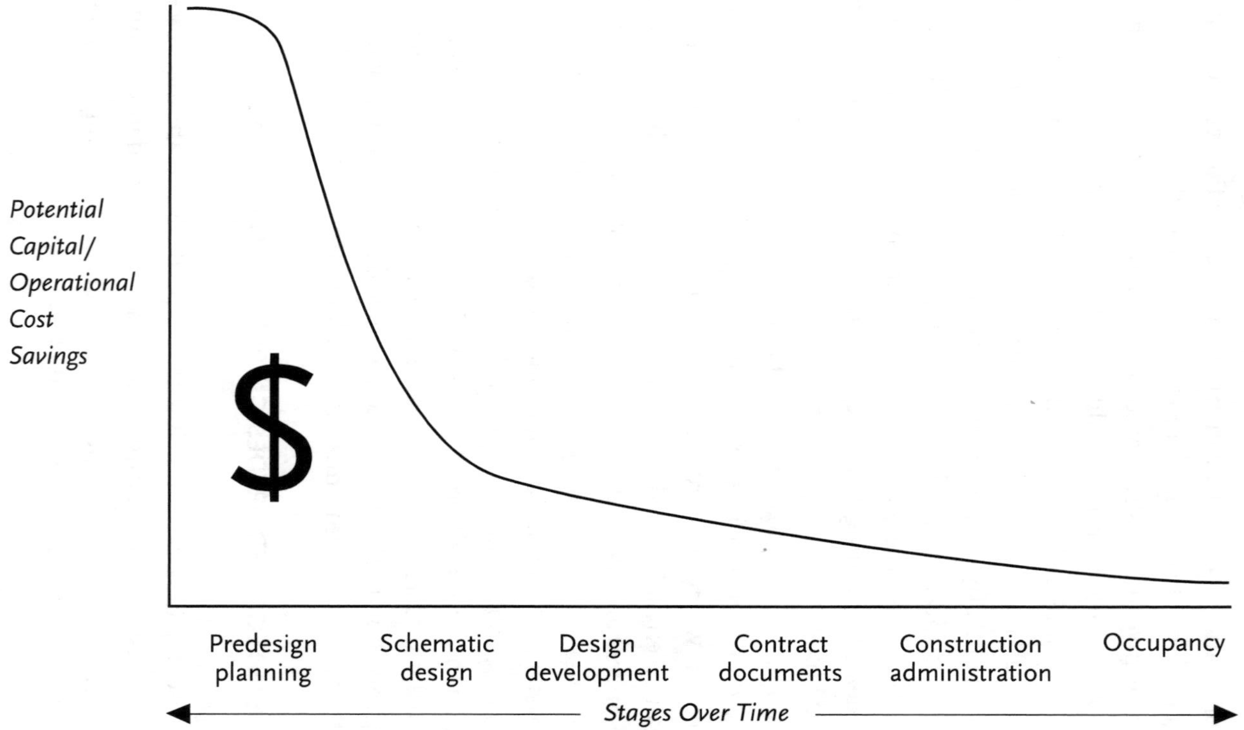

FIGURE 1.4 THE INTEGRATED PREDESIGN PLANNING PROCESS

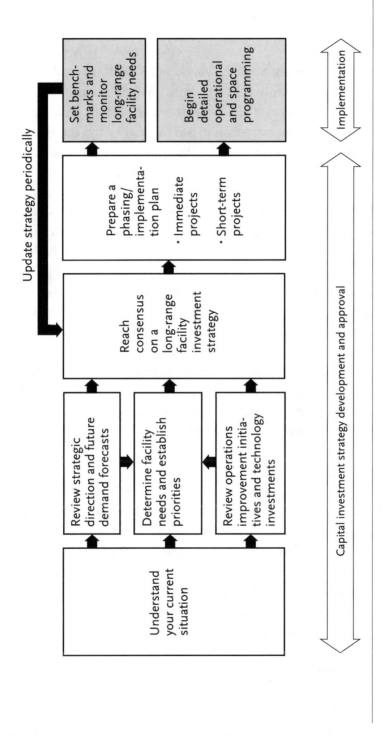

2. *Implementation*: this includes the detailed operational and space programming for designated projects and the establishment of benchmarks to monitor long-range facility needs as the strategy is periodically updated.

Capital Investment Strategy Development and Approval

The predesign process begins with the collection of baseline facility data and a review of the organization's current situation, including campus access and circulation, bed utilization and configuration, space allocation and layout, and infrastructure issues. Current market dynamics, workload trends, future vision, and projected demand are also reviewed and incorporated into the facility planning process, along with the organization's institutionwide and service-line-specific operations improvement initiatives. Planned technology investments are also concurrently reviewed and coordinated with the facility planning process.

Existing and future space need is documented and compared with current space allocation. At this point, future facility needs must be determined, priorities must be established, and consensus must be reached on a long-range facility investment strategy. Once the long-range facility investment strategy, or "road map," is defined, it can be divided or categorized into immediate, short-term, and long-range projects, which are assigned corresponding capital requirements that are sequenced over a multiyear period.

Implementation

With the phasing/implementation plan in hand, detailed operational (functional) and space programming can begin for those projects that are identified as immediate priorities, along with short-term projects for which planning needs to begin so that they can be completed within a two- to five-year planning horizon. Benchmarks are established for long-range projects; these benchmarks can be monitored over time and incorporated into the ongoing predesign planning process as the facility investment strategy is updated periodically.

THE PREDESIGN PLANNING TEAM

A facility planning committee or task force needs to be assembled and is typically led by the chief executive officer (CEO), chief operating officer (COO), or another designated senior executive within the organization. It may also be led by an outside consultant who has unique expertise in predesign planning. At the predesign planning stage, the facility planning committee generally includes the members of the existing management team and representatives from the medical staff and the building committee of the board. In addition, the organization's facility manager should be part of the team. The committee structure will ultimately reflect the organization's culture (top-down approach or bottom-up approach) but should not become overly large. A group of 9 to 12 members is manageable and provides a sufficient diversity of representation. The team will generally meet on a monthly basis but may meet more often, depending on the unique issues at hand.

Bringing a design architect or construction manager on board at the onset of the predesign planning stage is not necessary. Using an architect or facility planning consultant who is focused exclusively on predesign planning is desirable and prevents the potential conflict of interest associated with having the predesign planning process led by the firm that will ultimately be charged with the design or construction (and compensated at a percentage of the project cost). This is particularly relevant during the detailed operational and space programming phase.

If the organization has an "architect of record" (who often resides in the community, has had a long-term relationship with the organization, and has extensive knowledge of the physical plant), then this individual should be considered a valuable member of the predesign planning team.

Establishing the role of the committee is vital. The facility planning committee is typically responsible for prequalifying and selecting external consultants, reviewing and validating baseline data, confirming and challenging perceptions regarding facility deficiencies, and validating institutionwide and service-line-specific operational assumptions. The committee will also be responsible for translating the organization's vision into facility needs and priorities as well as for shaping the organization's long-range facility investment strategy. Once consensus is reached on this strategy, the committee needs to communicate it to the rest of the organization. In particular, the designated nursing and medical staff representatives must be able to educate their respective constituencies and act as emissaries to communicate and promote the benefits of the plan.

In some cases, specific feasibility studies may need to be conducted as part of the predesign planning stage and may require additional consultants, depending on the organization's in-house resources. These studies may include determination of whether a proposed project is financially, legally, or physically feasible. A design consultant or construction specialist may be asked to perform specific feasibility studies when a new or replacement healthcare facility is planned—for example, a site analysis—or when extensive facility renewal or replacement is required on a constrained site, and multiple architectural and engineering solutions may need to be evaluated. Such use of a design architect during the predesign planning process should not be confused with the subsequent stage of schematic design. It should be made clear to the selected design, engineering, or construction consultants that their work during the predesign planning stage is not a guarantee of future involvement in the subsequent design and construction of the proposed building project.

The facility planning committee is usually charged with prequalifying and selecting the design architect, construction manager, and other specialty consultants at the end of the predesign planning stage.

Once all predesign planning activities have been accomplished and the organization is ready to start the next stage—schematic design— the following books may be consulted as a reference:

- *The Non-Architect's Guide to Major Capital Projects—Planning, Designing, and Delivering New Buildings* by Phillip Waite. This book addresses the design and construction process, contracting approaches, and the project delivery team. See reference list.

- *Launching a Healthcare Capital Project* by John Kemper. This book is a good resource when a new or replacement hospital project is planned. See reference list.

NOTE

1. MBIA Insurance Corporation letter to Medicare Payment Advisory Commission (MedPac), January 2002.

REFERENCES

American Hospital Association (AHA). 2002. *Cracks in the Foundation—Averting a Crisis in America's Hospitals*. Chicago: Health Forum, an American Hospital Association Company.

American Hospital Association (AHA) and Lewin Group. 2004. *TrendWatch Chartbook 2004: Trends Affecting Hospitals and Health Systems*. Chicago: American Hospital Association.

DeNavas-Walt, C., B. D. Proctor, and B. J. Mills. 2004. *Income, Poverty, and Health Insurance Coverage in the United States*: 2003. U.S. Census Bureau Report P60–226. [Online information; retrieved 7/21/05.] www.census.gov/hhes/www/income.html.

Hayward, C. 1995. "Avoiding Construction of Inappropriate Health Care Facilities." In *Plant, Technology, and Safety Management Series: Health Facility Design and Construction* 1 (1995 Series), 19–23. Oakbrook Terrace, IL: Joint Commission on Accreditation of Healthcare Organizations.

————. 2004. *SpaceMed—A Space Planning Guide for Healthcare Facilities*. Ann Arbor, MI: Hayward & Associates, LLC. [Online information; retrieved 7/21/05.] www.space-med.com.

Herzlinger, R. 2002. "Let's Put Consumers in Charge of Health Care." *Harvard Business Review* 80 (7): 44–55.

Ingenix and Healthcare Financial Management Association (HFMA). 2002. *Almanac of Hospital Financial and Operating Indicators 1994–2002*. Columbus, OH: Center for Healthcare Industry Performance Studies.

InterStudy Publications. 2004. *InterStudy Competitive Edge: HMO Industry Report Fall 2004*. St. Paul, MN: Decision Resources, Inc.

Jaklevic, M. C. 2002. "Mauled by the Bear: Investment Losses and Not-for-Profits Have Taken a Big Bite Out of the Bottom Line, But Hospitals Are Staying in Stocks for the Long Haul." *Modern Healthcare* 32 (44): 34–37.

Kemper, J. 2004. *Launching a Healthcare Capital Project*. Chicago: Health Administration Press.

Kohn, L. T., J. M. Corrigan, and M. S. Donaldson (eds.). 2000. *To Err Is Human: Building a Safer Health System*. Washington, DC: Institute of Medicine, National Academies Press.

The National Center for Health Workforce Analysis. 2002. *Projected Supply, Demand, and Shortages of Registered Nurses: 2000–2020*. Washington, DC: U.S. Department of Health and Human Services, Health Resources and Services Administration, Bureau of Health Professions.

PricewaterhouseCoopers. 2001. "Survey of Hospitals and Health Systems." In *Cracks in the Foundation—Averting a Crisis in America's Hospitals*. [Online information; retrieved 7/21/05.] http://www.aha.org/aha/advocacy-grassroots/advocacy/advocacy/content/cracksreprint08-02.pdf.

Waite, P. S. 2005. *The Non-Architect's Guide to Major Capital Projects: Planning, Designing, and Delivering New Buildings*. Ann Arbor, MI: Society for College and University Planning.

CHAPTER TWO

Understanding Your Current Facility

COLLECTING AND ANALYZING data on your current facility is the first step in preparing a long-range capital investment strategy. Knowing your facility's current site access and circulation, layout and configuration, space allocation, and physical condition will allow you to identify key issues and to establish priorities. Assessing the success of a major renovation or construction project is very difficult without a thorough understanding of the baseline conditions.

Key questions to ask when analyzing the facility may include the following:

- How much land do we occupy, and how do our customers access our site and facilities?

- What type of space do we have, and where is it located?

- How many beds do we have, and how are they organized?

- How many and what types of diagnostic and treatment spaces do we use? How much space are we currently using?

- What ongoing investment will be required for infrastructure upgrading and ongoing maintenance of our physical plant?

WORKING FROM THE OUTSIDE INWARD

Evaluating the current facility should begin with a review of overall property boundaries and site access points. Designated campus circulation routes and corresponding parking areas should be identified by type of traffic, such as emergency vehicles, service trucks, patients, and visitors. The number of parking spaces available by type (if restricted) should also be tabulated. In addition, potential areas for physical expansion and expansion constraints, such as underground utilities, easements, and covenants, should be identified. Key building entrances should also be noted.

Every healthcare campus must accommodate the flow of a variety of customers, including patients, visitors, staff, and physicians; ambulance and emergency traffic; and service traffic. Identifying and tracking the different types of circulation facilitates a wayfinding assessment. *Wayfinding* begins with the customer's arrival on the campus, and it involves signage and visual cues to assist customers in identifying the appropriate building entrance, finding parking if necessary, and arriving at the desired service location.

Expediting campus access for emergency vehicles and emergent patients arriving by private vehicle is particularly important in designing a campus that facilitates wayfinding. Outpatients may be directed to a medical office building, a hospital-based clinic, or a diagnostic area for a routine visit or procedure. They may also be directed to a surgery or special procedure center, after which they may require an extended recovery or admission. Most healthcare campuses also accommodate outpatients with chronic conditions who require recurring care, such as physical therapy or dialysis patients, and may need to navigate the hospital campus frequently. Unless admitted through the ED, most patients today arrive at the hospital as an outpatient and are generally admitted post-procedure.

In addition to patient traffic, the healthcare campus must accommodate visitors and family members who may arrive separately or who may drop off a patient, park, and then reunite with the patient. Hospital employees and their vehicles must also be given a well-defined circulation system, and the same should be available to physicians who need to park and access either their clinical workplace or support service areas such as medical records. A separate circulation system should be provided for service traffic, such as delivery trucks and trash pick-up, to access the loading dock. Service traffic should not be visible to patients and visitors and should certainly not impede ambulance and emergency traffic.

ALL SPACE IS NOT THE SAME

First, an understanding of the different types of space within a health-care facility, their general characteristics, the factors influencing space need, and current space planning trends (as summarized in Table 2.1) is necessary. Different types, or categories, of space may have varying building-code-compliance requirements, renovation or construction costs, and reuse potential.

Inpatient Nursing Units

Based on my experience, these units generally occupy 35 percent to 40 percent of the total usable space in a community hospital. This type of space must comply with the most stringent hospital building codes, because it is occupied by extended length-of-stay patients who are not ambulatory. In an era of fluctuating demand, nurse staffing shortages, and limited access to capital, the management of this large space is a significant issue for most healthcare organizations. Inpatient nursing units represent a major portion of an organization's revenue base (and operational costs), and the construction or renovation of inpatient nursing units is expensive compared to that of other types of space.

The layout of a typical inpatient floor is based on a common patient-room module that includes a fixed plumbing chase to support a contiguous patient toilet/shower room. Building codes require that all patient rooms have windows to admit natural light. Patient rooms are accessed from a horizontal circulation corridor (which is eight feet wide at a minimum) that leads to elevator lobbies and stairwells that in turn provide vertical circulation to the rest of the facility. Patient rooms are supplemented by various support spaces (which do not require natural light) that are placed in an inner-core area.

Patient acuity and length of stay are the primary factors that affect the number of beds, the size of the patient room, and the corresponding support space. Higher-acuity patients or extended-stay patients require additional space. Larger patient rooms are required for sicker patients who may require emergency intervention or treatments that involve additional equipment and staff. Although they do not require

TABLE 2.1 CHARACTERISTICS OF DIFFERENT TYPES OF SPACE IN A HEALTHCARE FACILITY

Category of Space	Facility Characteristics	Space Drivers	Current Trends
Inpatient nursing units	• Modular construction • Limited flexibility for cost-effective reuse • Most stringent code requirements due to patient acuity/extended length of stay • Revenue generating	• Patient care delivery model • Acuity and length of stay • Unit size • Type of patient accommodations • Technology/operational systems • Facility layout/design • Desired amenities	• Increasing patient acuity • Expanding information technology • Larger, autonomous patient care units (e.g., hospital within a hospital) • Flexible design for alternate levels of care • Facility layout designed to optimize scarce nursing personnel • Demand for private rooms
Diagnostic and treatment	• Generally accommodates inpatients and outpatients, unless outpatient volume justifies redundant equipment, staff, and space • More stringent code requirements with inpatient occupancy • Some modalities are expensive to build and have unique architectural design requirements (e.g., operating rooms, interventional imaging, MR); other modalities use miniaturized, mobile equipment • Rapidly changing technology • Revenue generating (outpatient primarily)	• Organizational structure • Patient mix • Technology/operational concepts • Throughput of equipment • Average versus peak workloads • Scheduling patterns • Number of physician/administrative offices • Recruitment promises	• Rapid advances in technology and melding/blurring of modalities • Extended hours of operation to optimize equipment utilization • Optimizing flexibility and sharing of resources (e.g., equipment, staff, space) • Miniaturized, more mobile equipment • Shift to point-of-care services • Networking with physician offices • Advances in telemedicine (e.g., patient remote from specialty physician/technician) • Increased "stat" and 24/7 requests to facilitate throughput and shorten length of stay
Customer service and amenities	• First point of entry/contact for patients and their families • Typically includes a variety of "departments" and amenities (e.g., lobbies/lounges) • Cost of space varies with amenities desired	• Institutional policy • Departmental/organizational structure • Overall traffic volume and circulation/flow patterns • Scope of retail activities	• Replication of "hotel" reception desk (hub and spoke) model • Focus on first impression/image • Operational restructuring around needs of customer

Clinical support	• Minimal patient traffic • Specialized design considerations • Increased use of robotics (e.g., laboratory, pharmacy) • Shift to point-of-care services	• Equipment/technology more critical than workload volume • Staffing on the day (primary) shift	• Increased automation and use of robotics, barcoding, etc. • Unbundling services to less expensive space
Physician practice	• Ambulatory patient traffic • Less expensive construction • Significant parking requirements • Demand depends on who pays for space	• Scope of diagnostic procedures/treatments • Workload and scheduling patterns • Shared use versus exclusive use • Number and location of physician administrative offices	• Time-share concept, with more efficient scheduling of exam/treatment space • Extended hours of operation • Competition for outpatients with convenient access and contiguous parking • Variable impact of reimbursement on service locations and facility configuration
Administrative offices	• Typically generic office space and non-revenue producing • Limited patient/visitor traffic • Least stringent code requirements • Less costly to build/renovate	• Organizational structure • Staff on primary (day) shift • Communication/information technology • Shared use versus exclusive use	• Reorganization of traditional departments to optimize sharing of resources • Creation of generic office space and consolidation in less expensive space
Building support	• No patient traffic • Generally open, industrial space • Least costly construction • Inpatient units are primary "users" • Services should be opaque to customers	• Primarily hospital beds • Organizational structure and operational concepts • Equipment/technology • Make, buy, sell decisions	• Shift to point-of-care and on-demand services • Unbundling of services into less expensive space (e.g., service building) • Advances in technology (e.g., robotics, barcoding, RFID) • Outsourcing

larger patient rooms, inpatient units for extended lengths of stay—for example, rehabilitation units and skilled nursing units—must provide additional support space for group dining, therapy, and family visitation, according to current guidelines (AIA and FGI 2001).

The size of a specific nursing unit, which is defined as a group of patient rooms that shares a central nursing station and support space (along with a single nurse manager and unit clerk), is also influenced by the mix of private versus semiprivate patient rooms, planned operational and technical support systems, and the level of amenities desired. However, the optimal number of beds on a given nursing unit or floor is related to the modular divisibility of the total number of beds. For example, a 32-bed nursing unit can be divided into subunits of 4, 6, or 8 beds, or it can be divided into two subunits of 16 beds. Flexible designs are being developed that can accommodate alternate staffing patterns and levels of care either by shift or over time to minimize future renovation if the patient population changes.

Because of the modular nature of an inpatient unit, this type of space poses a challenge when conversion to non-inpatient use is considered. Reassignment for an alternate functional use either results in inefficient space utilization, when the space is reused without physical reconfiguration, or involves high renovation costs, when walls (and utility chases) are moved. Because the rigid column/bay spacing and numerous fixed utility chases often make major reconfiguration cost prohibitive, most organizations find that they are limited to infrastructure upgrades and cosmetic renovations of nursing units.

When inpatient space is either no longer needed or has become functionally obsolete, a common practice is to redeploy or downgrade the space for administrative offices. However, compared to building or leasing space in an office building, this practice requires more space to house a given number of offices. Higher operational costs also result, because the surplus space—for example, wider corridors and toilet/shower rooms—still must be cleaned, maintained, insured, and secured.

Diagnostic and Treatment

This space typically accommodates inpatients and outpatients. When outpatient workload volumes are sufficient to justify redundant resources—equipment, staff, and space—or when necessitated by strategic (market) partnering dynamics, dedicated or freestanding outpatient facilities are developed. Procedure rooms may need to be designed for sophisticated digital equipment with unique design and environmental requirements—for example, lead shielding or reinforced floors—or they may require no more than an exam table, sink, and storage cabinetry to support a small piece of portable equipment.

As with inpatient nursing units, diagnostic and treatment services are a source of revenue and are therefore frequent targets of expansion when incremental demand is anticipated. In addition to the current and projected workloads, the patient mix, level of technology, operational concepts, throughput of the equipment, scheduling patterns, and overall organizational structure all affect the amount of space needed. The fulfillment of recruitment promises to physicians also frequently drives the type of equipment and amount of space allocated.

Because of rapid advances in new technology, minimally invasive diagnostic and treatment capabilities, the shift to point-of-care services, and the blending and melding of some of the traditional imaging modalities, healthcare organizations are increasingly focusing on long-range flexibility when constructing diagnostic and treatment space. The trend is toward creation of generic "large" and "small" procedure rooms that can accommodate varying equipment over time and are supported by shared patient intake, preparation, and recovery areas.

Customer Service and Amenities

Such space is used by multiple departments and staff involved in assisting the patient, family members, and others with navigating the array of healthcare services both on and off site. Space in this category generally includes areas for reception, admitting and registration, central scheduling, cashiering, insurance verification, physician referrals, and various similar services. This category of space also includes amenities such as lobbies, lounges, gift shops, cafes, and libraries/resource centers that may be found in any hospitality facility—a hotel, for example. Unfortunately, many acute care hospitals still organize these services in line with their traditional departments rather than around the needs of the patients and other customers. Many of these departments are located on the first floor of the healthcare facility (which is prime real estate), even though only a small number of staff actually have face-to-face contact with patients and their families.

Space need is influenced primarily by the organization of these services and the number of staff who require workstations.

Institutional policies regarding the amount and scope of amenities to be provided and the ambiance to be achieved also affect the space allocation in any given facility. Key trends include replicating the hotel reception-desk concept (hub-and-spoke model) to enhance customer satisfaction and creating a positive first impression upon initial entry into the facility.

Support space for other customers may include staff lockers and lounges, fitness facilities, and day care centers for employees' children.

Clinical Support

This space includes the clinical laboratory, pharmacy, central sterile processing, and similar services that, although unique to a healthcare facility, do not accommodate patient traffic as diagnostic and treatment services do. Space need, physical configuration, and location are determined primarily by the type of equipment and technology deployed rather than by actual workload. Significant developments in automation and robotics, barcoding, and information management have drastically altered the way this type of space is planned today. With efficient delivery systems in place for specimens, medications, and instruments, to name a few, many of these clinical support services are being relocated to less expensive, industrial-style space.

Physician Practice

This space typically consists of a patient reception (intake) area; a large number of identical exam rooms; a smaller number of offices, consultation rooms, and special-procedure rooms; and accompanying support space. Construction of physician practice space, which is exclusively used by outpatients, is less expensive than other types of patient care space described above. Physician practice space may be located in a medical office building (either freestanding or connected to an acute care hospital), be collocated with diagnostic and treatment services in a comprehensive ambulatory care center, or be part of an institute or "center of excellence" that is organized along a specific product line such as cardiology, cancer, orthopedics, or geriatrics.

Physicians may own their office space, lease dedicated space, participate in a time-share arrangement, or work in hospital-sponsored clinics. The size and configuration of the space will vary, depending on the medical practice model and scheduling patterns, the workload volumes and exam room turnaround, and the scope of diagnostic and treatment procedures.

Physician practice space is often located in one or more freestanding buildings on a healthcare campus, which is typical of specialists, or distributed throughout the community, which is typical of primary care physicians, to provide contiguous patient parking and convenient access. Because most physicians use relatively generic space, time-share concepts are becoming increasingly popular as a way to optimize space utilization and to minimize the rental and operational costs born by the individual physician or group practice.

Administrative Offices

This space is used by many hospital departments involved in the administration and management of the organization. Regardless of the department assignment, this space generally includes a mix of private offices, enclosed or semi-enclosed cubicles, and open workstations to accommodate different hierarchies of staff as dictated by the organizational structure. Patient and family traffic is rare in such spaces. Much of the administrative space is occupied only during standard business hours, and the number of staff and the organizational structure dictate the amount of space required. Operational reengineering and advancements in information technology in the past decade have reduced the number of administrative staff not involved in direct patient care. At the same time, every new program requires some amount of office space, and the consolidation of existing services often results in the need for a larger block of space in a single location.

Building Support

This space is required for those services that support any large, industrial or hospitality complex, and it includes materials management, environmental services, and food services. Space for these services should function efficiently in the background and be opaque to patients and visitors. These services use open, industrial-style space that, with the exception of the kitchen, is perhaps the least costly space to construct and renovate, assuming that it is not integrated with the hospital chassis such that it must be built or maintained to more stringent hospital codes. Kitchen space, on the other hand, is among the most expensive space per square foot to construct on the healthcare campus.

The need for building support space is primarily driven by the number of inpatients; the equipment and technology to be deployed; and the decisions by the organization to make, buy, or sell these services. The unbundling of these services into inexpensive, industrial-style space and the increased use of automated distribution systems, robotics, and electronic materials management and inventory systems also affect the size and configuration of the space.

Other Space

"Other" categories may include research and education space. Such space is an integral part of most academic medical centers but not commonly found in community hospitals, with the exception of space for clinical trials and central or decentralized conference and training facilities. The need for research space is driven by program funding and recruiting promises. The amount of education space will depend on the specific educational programs, scheduling patterns, and typical number of participants. In-service education on the healthcare campus is being redefined with the increased use of distance learning concepts such as video conferencing, Internet meetings and presentations, and self-directed learning. At the same time, the proliferation of new technology, particularly information technology, is creating new demands for in-service education. Some healthcare organizations, however, opt to lease space (as needed) at local community centers, hotels, or schools in lieu of constructing large meeting rooms or an auditorium for infrequent use.

DIFFERENTIATING BETWEEN NET SPACE AND GROSS SPACE

Frequent misunderstandings arise when hospital leaders, department staff, planners, and architects confuse *net square feet* with *gross square feet*. As shown in Figure 2.1, net square feet (NSF) refers to the inside, wall-to-wall dimensions within a room or area and represents the actual usable space. The total of the net square feet of all usable rooms and areas within a department is referred to as the *department net square feet* (DNSF). However, the most common term used in facility master planning is *department gross square feet* (DGSF), which represents the "footprint" of the specific department. DGSF includes the space occupied by internal circulation corridors, walls and partitions, and minor utility columns, in addition to the usable NSF within the department. DGSF excludes common areas such as shared public corridors and lobbies, elevator banks, stairwells, major mechanical spaces, the space occupied by the building's exterior wall, central toilet facilities, housekeeping, equipment storage, and other shared space.

FIGURE 2.1 COMPARISON OF NET SQUARE FEET AND GROSS SQUARE FEET

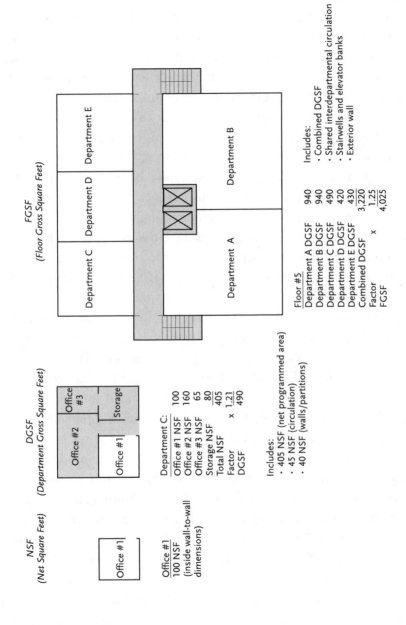

NSF
(Net Square Feet)

DGSF
(Department Gross Square Feet)

FGSF
(Floor Gross Square Feet)

Office #1
100 NSF
(inside wall-to-wall dimensions)

Department C:
Office #1 NSF	100
Office #2 NSF	160
Office #3 NSF	65
Storage NSF	80
Total NSF	405
Factor	x 1.21
DGSF	490

Includes:
- 405 NSF (net programmed area)
- 45 NSF (circulation)
- 40 NSF (walls/partitions)

Floor #5
Department A DGSF	940
Department B DGSF	940
Department C DGSF	490
Department D DGSF	420
Department E DGSF	430
Combined DGSF	3,220
Factor	x 1.25
FGSF	4,025

Includes:
- Combined DGSF
- Shared interdepartmental circulation
- Stairwells and elevator banks
- Exterior wall

Source: Hayward, C. 2005. *SpaceMed—A Space Planning Guide for Healthcare Facilities.* Ann Arbor, MI: Hayward & Associates, LLC. [Online information; retrieved 7/21/05.] www.space-med.com.

To convert the sum of all net spaces to an estimate of the actual department footprint, a *net-to-department gross space conversion factor* is used. The estimated DGSF is used to test the feasibility of different facility configuration options during facility master planning and to estimate renovation costs prior to design.

Net-to-department gross space conversion factors generally range from 1.20 to 1.50. Large, open spaces—for example, those usually planned for building support services such as materials management and environmental services—would have a lower factor because of a limited number of walls and partitions and minimal internal corridors. A surgery suite would have a larger factor to account for numerous and variously sized rooms that must be connected by eight-foot-wide corridors to accommodate patients' stretchers. The factor for a specific functional area will also vary depending on whether new construction is planned (lower factor) or if the function is to be retrofitted into existing space with specific design constraints (higher factor). Constraints, such as the shape of the existing building envelope, minimal bay width and unusual column spacing, and fixed mechanical spaces and pipe shafts, may require a greater amount of DGSF to accommodate the same amount of NSF than in new construction.

Additional factors are used to estimate the overall size of a floor and the building footprint to develop early (predesign) construction cost estimates. An additional 20 percent to 30 percent (or a factor of 1.20 to 1.30) is generally used to arrive at an estimate for the *floor gross square feet* (FGSF) that accounts for the common areas on the floor. To estimate the total *building gross square feet* (BGSF), an additional 8 percent to 12 percent (or a factor of 1.08 to 1.12) may be required to allow for major mechanical spaces and a central power plant, depending on the scope of the project and existing capacity. Larger factors are required to accommodate unique design features such as atriums and courtyards. Ultimately, the actual design will determine the final space requirements. However, if the eventual design affords very large net-to-gross space conversion factors and calls for no special architectural features, the overall efficiency of the design should be questioned—for example, look for redundant corridors. Dividing the total BGSF by the actual usable space, or NSF, is often referred to as the *building efficiency ratio* and is expressed as a percentage.

To confuse the matter further, universities often use the term *assignable square feet* to describe all rooms and areas that are available for assignment to an individual program, department, or user. They then use the term *net assignable (or usable) area* to describe the combined total of the NSF and the common or shared areas.

Yet again, a slightly different set of terms is used by commercial realtors that need to be understood if a healthcare organization wishes to lease space off campus. The Building Owners and Managers Association (BOMA) International applies the term *usable square feet* to define the footprint of the space that is assigned to the tenant under their direct control, and then it applies a factor for the tenant's share of the common areas to arrive at the *rentable square feet* on which the tenant will pay rent. In typical multitenant, multistory buildings, the common area factor can range from 14 percent to 16 percent. In smaller buildings with fewer amenities and smaller lobbies, the factor ranges from 10 percent to 12 percent. The International Facilities Management Association (IFMA) has developed its own definition of rentable square feet, which is also used by facility managers to allocate or charge-back square footage to specific departments.

Although this discussion of net and gross space may seem tedious, misunderstandings among members of the planning team can be disastrous, because the DGSF is typically 20 percent to 50 percent higher than the DNSF. For example, confusing department *net* square feet with department *gross* square feet can deem certain facility configuration options feasible when they are not or can result in inaccurate early cost estimates. Physicians and clinical department managers may ask their peers at other institutions for comparative space information and receive the "square feet" with no indication of how it was calculated, and may then use this information to demand that their existing space be enlarged. Knowledge of how space allocation is calculated also eliminates surprises when leasing space off site.

NSF and DGSF used for facility planning should not be confused with other methods of space measurement used by finance to account for charge-backs to individual departments, cost reimbursement, asset tracking, and so on.

BED ALLOCATION AND ORGANIZATION

Any facility assessment of an acute care hospital should begin with an inventory and analysis of the inpatient nursing units. Inpatient nursing units are modular in design and vary in the number and type of patient rooms (private, semiprivate), configuration of the patient toilet/shower facilities, and the total DGSF used to support the specific number of beds. The following data should be collected for each inpatient nursing unit:

- Bed licensure by category of beds, acuity, or service line, according to the specific state regulatory requirements

- Current number of staffed inpatient beds on which the daily/monthly census and occupancy are calculated

- Number of staffed beds in private rooms versus double or semiprivate rooms (or multiple-bed rooms)

- Total number of staffed patient rooms by nursing unit, including private and multiple-bed rooms.

In addition, the *design capacity* of each nursing unit should be identified based on physical inspection of the unit or current architectural drawings, or both. The design capacity refers to the total number of beds that could be deployed for inpatient care with minimal renovation, regardless of the number of beds actually staffed at any given time. Additional beds and rooms that may be counted as part of the design capacity may include patient rooms temporarily used as offices or storage rooms (but where the headwalls and utilities are still intact) or smaller, semiprivate rooms used as private rooms during low-census periods. The nursing units should be further aggregated by the type of beds they contain—for example, general medical or surgical, intensive care, maternity, or psychiatric. This helps the planning team to understand which beds are generally interchangeable such that they can be readily reassigned from one service line to another versus those that are designed as unique units for a specific patient population. Additional information on evaluating inpatient bed capacity is provided in Chapter 5 along with an example of an inpatient bed inventory (see Figure 5.2).

SPACE LOCATION AND CONFIGURATION

With a thorough understanding of the various types of space within a healthcare facility, one of the key steps in developing a facility planning database is to document the functional layout of your current facilities by identifying where different categories of space are located. Simple floor plans that identify department locations by floor, building, or wing need to be assembled, as shown in Figure 2.2. Most organizations have "as is" architectural drawings in an electronic format, which can be used to "block out" existing department boundaries. The newly generated department location or *block* floor plans are typically color coded according to the category of space and are reduced to a manageable size. Building section, or "stacking," diagrams, as shown in Figure 2.3, are also useful communication tools.

MAJOR DIAGNOSTIC AND TREATMENT SPACES

In addition to the number of staffed beds, an inventory of major diagnostic and treatment spaces will be key to evaluating your current facility capacity, which is addressed in Chapter 5. The major diagnostic and treatment spaces—rooms, cubicles, or open stretcher bays—that generate revenue and affect the workload that can be accommodated at your organization include the following:

- ED treatment rooms and/or bays

- Surgical operating rooms, such as open heart, general, and cysto, and patient preparation bays and recovery bays

- Labor, delivery, operating/caesarian section rooms; LDR rooms

- Imaging procedure rooms such as x-ray, computerized tomography (CT), magnetic resonance imaging (MRI), and radiation therapy

- Interventional procedure rooms such as cardiac catheterization and angiography

- Other procedure rooms with fixed equipment such as endoscopy

- Exam and procedure rooms with mobile equipment such as ultrasound, echocardiography, and electrocardiography (EKG)

- Exam and treatment rooms, typically found in clinics

FIGURE 2.2 EXAMPLE OF A DEPARTMENT LOCATION DIAGRAM (FLOOR PLAN)

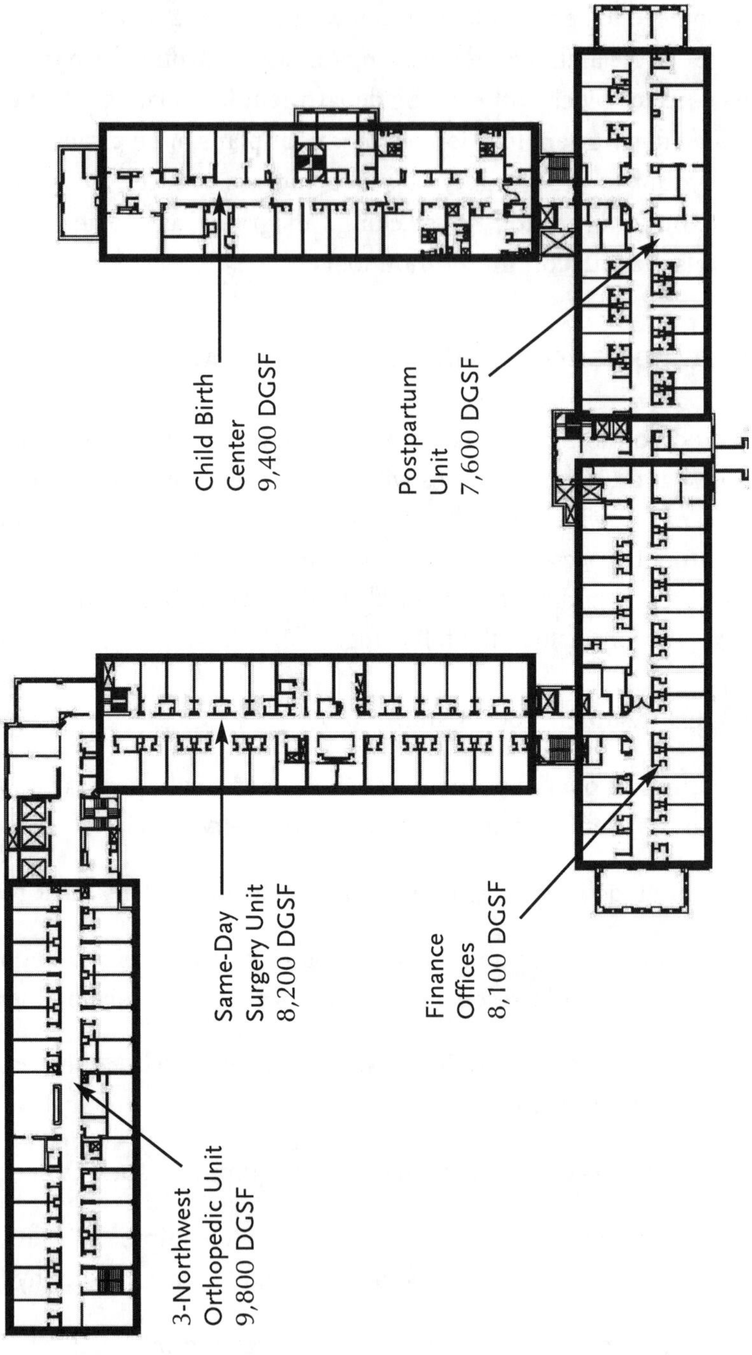

Child Birth
Center
9,400 DGSF

Postpartum
Unit
7,600 DGSF

Same-Day
Surgery Unit
8,200 DGSF

Finance
Offices
8,100 DGSF

3-Northwest
Orthopedic Unit
9,800 DGSF

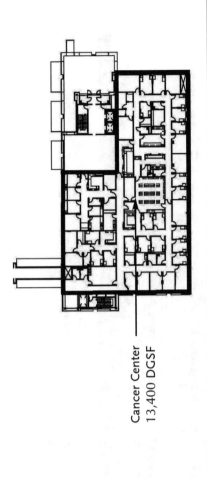

Cancer Center
13,400 DGSF

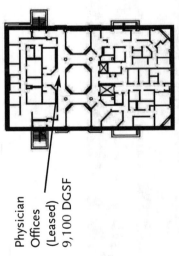

Physician
Offices
(Leased)
9,100 DGSF

FIGURE 2.3 EXAMPLE OF A BUILDING SECTION DIAGRAM

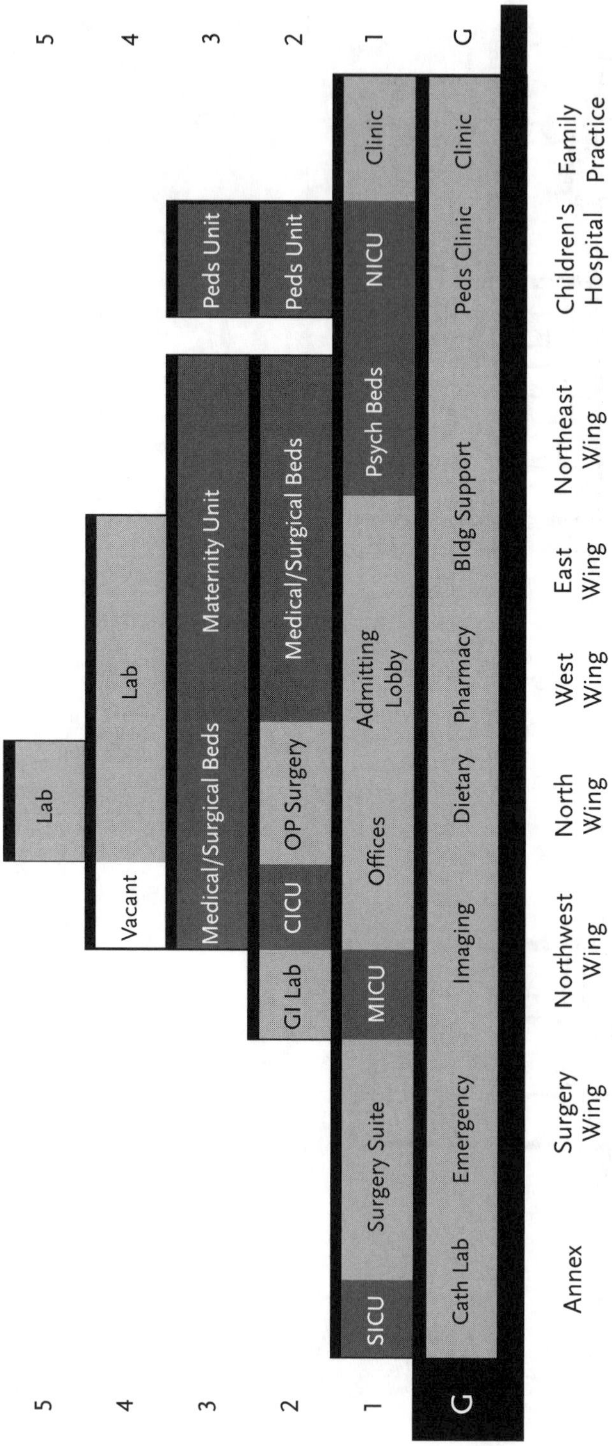

Floor levels (left axis): 5, 4, 3, 2, 1, G

	Annex	Surgery Wing	Northwest Wing	North Wing	West Wing	East Wing	Northeast Wing	Children's Hospital	Family Practice
5				Lab					
4		Lab		Vacant	Lab				
3			Medical/Surgical Beds	Medical/Surgical Beds		Maternity Unit		Peds Unit	
2			GI Lab	CICU	OP Surgery	Medical/Surgical Beds		Peds Unit	
1	SICU	Surgery Suite	MICU	Offices	Admitting Lobby	Psych Beds		NICU	Clinic
G		Cath Lab	Emergency	Imaging	Dietary	Pharmacy	Bldg Support	Peds Clinic	Clinic

- Other procedure, treatment, or recovery bays typically used for chemotherapy, medical procedures, phlebotomy, and physical therapy

For major imaging and interventional procedure rooms, the current type of equipment and its acquisition date should be identified. As is discussed in Chapter 5, the age and sophistication of the equipment may have a significant impact on its capacity to handle a given workload.

SPACE ALLOCATION

Having two architects or facility managers measure the same building and arrive at the same net and gross square footage number is virtually impossible unless there is agreement on the method of measurement and a clear definition of what is included and excluded, as described previously. The use of computer-aided drafting (CAD) supported by field measurements is far more accurate than trying to scale from old architectural drawings that may not reflect "as is" versus "as built" conditions. Once the floor plans are in an electronic format, the footprint of each department can be electronically defined and measured. The resulting inventory of current DGSF can then be organized by major functional category of space and the space tabulated by department, floor level, and building as appropriate.

From my experience, the typical distribution of assignable space (DGSF) in a community hospital is shown in Figure 2.4 (excluding physician practice space). The ranges represent variations in patient accommodations (private versus semiprivate inpatient room mix); service consolidation versus decentralization; on-site versus off-site service locations; and institutional policies regarding the scope of patient, visitor, and staff amenities.

Why all the emphasis on these functional categories of space? There are two primary reasons. First, organizing space in this manner facilitates cost effective space reconfiguration, because the space occupied by a department within a functional category can be more readily and cost effectively redeployed for use by another department in that category. Second, the grouping of departments that have similar facility requirements often exposes new opportunities for the sharing or cross-utilization of space between organizational entities.

FIGURE 2.4 TYPICAL COMMUNITY HOSPITAL SPACE ALLOCATION (DEPARTMENT GROSS SQUARE FEET)

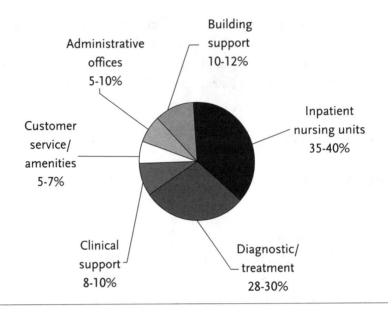

The DGSF for an inpatient nursing unit should include the eight-foot circulation corridors within the nursing units, even though they are used for public egress. However, central elevator lobbies, elevator banks, stairwells, and major mechanical space should be excluded from the DGSF for an inpatient nursing unit.

MAJOR PHYSICAL PLANT AND INFRASTRUCTURE ISSUES

First, let's address how information about the condition of the physical plant and building infrastructure is used during the facility master planning process. The primary reason for a detailed engineering evaluation is to identify code noncompliances and other critical physical plant issues that could affect the viability of the business enterprise. Second, infrastructure deficiencies must be identified, and costs and a timetable developed for their correction, for capital budgeting. Every healthcare organization should include the ongoing upgrading of its infrastructure and physical plant as one of its long-range facility investment strategies. Like any other business, healthcare organizations need to continually maintain and update their physical plants and retool their facilities to meet changing demand and new technology. The ongoing cost of infrastructure upgrading must be known as other construction or reconfiguration costs are identified. This ensures that adequate dollars are available for both over the multiyear planning period.

Physical plant and infrastructure upgrading issues will be more or less critical to the facility master planning effort, depending on the general age and condition of a medical center's facilities. An exhaustive and comprehensive engineering assessment may be undertaken that incorporates a detailed evaluation of all building systems, including structural, mechanical, plumbing, electrical, and fire safety. However, healthcare organizations should be cautious when embarking on this type of comprehensive and detailed assessment of the physical plant before a thorough analysis of the current functional layout, wayfinding issues, and future space need is undertaken. Buildings and wings have a tendency to become functionally obsolete for specific services before they become physically obsolete, and time and money may be saved if a more specific and targeted engineering assessment will suffice.

Hospital boards may face sticker shock when the results of an extensive engineering assessment are presented and the associated costs itemized. This is particularly distressing because the benefit of spending millions of dollars on infrastructure upgrading is not generally apparent to patients, physicians, and staff. Some board members may recall that the construction of the original hospital had cost less than the current dollars requested for a new power plant, electrical upgrading, elevator replacement, fire safety improvements, and the like. This frequently results in the question, how much would it cost to replace the existing hospital with new construction in lieu of spending so much money on upgrading the infrastructure?

SUMMARY OF BASELINE FACILITY PLANNING DATA

The following list summarizes the baseline facility planning data that are needed:

- Site plan that includes property boundaries, campus circulation routes, parking by type, and key building entrance points

- Department block floor plans

- Summary of inpatient beds and nursing units

- Identification of major diagnostic and treatment spaces,
  as well as the type and age of imaging equipment as applicable

- Space inventory in DGSF

- Identification of major infrastructure issues and remediation
  costs

NOTE

For additional reference, see Hayward, C. 2005. *SpaceMed—A Space Planning Guide for Healthcare Facilities*. Ann Arbor, MI: Hayward & Associates, LLC. [Online information; retrieved 7/21/05.] www.space-med.com.

REFERENCE

American Institute of Architects (AIA) and Facilities Guidelines Institute (FGI). 2001. *Guidelines for Design and Construction of Health Care Facilities*. Washington, DC: American Institute of Architects Press.

CHAPTER THREE

Defining Strategic Direction and Future Demand

I N HEALTHCARE STRATEGIC Planning: Approaches for the 21st Century, author Alan Zuckerman (1998) describes a four-stage strategic planning approach for healthcare organizations:

1. *Situation analysis* involves a review of the organization's mission, philosophy, and culture; an external assessment of the market structure and dynamics; an internal assessment of distinctive characteristics; and an evaluation of competitive position in the market.

2. *Strategic direction/vision* is where alternative futures, mission, vision, and key strategies are formulated.

3. *Strategy formulation* is where goals and objectives for the organization are established, particularly related to critical issues.

4. *Action planning* involves identifying the actions needed to implement the plan, such as the schedule, priorities, and resources.

Although this overall process is similar to that used to develop a long-range facility master plan (or capital investment strategy), most healthcare organizations use the term *strategic planning* to describe market planning with an increasing emphasis on surviving financially while fulfilling the organization's mission. The strategic (market) planning process logically precedes facility planning, assuming that business strategies must be in place and future demand must be forecasted before resources, such as facilities, equipment, and staff, can be defined. However, there are several benefits to integrating, or at least overlapping, these efforts.

UNDERSTANDING YOUR MARKET AND PATIENT POPULATION

An important component of strategic planning is an assessment of the organization's market and the socioeconomic characteristics of the service area population. Patients may have different perceptions and expectations depending on their age, sex, ethnicity, average income, education level, occupation, and so on. Although the patient population to be served by a healthcare organization may change over the life of the facilities, hospital leaders, facility planners, and architects should have a general understanding of the patient population for which their facilities are planned.

INTEGRATING FACILITY PLANNING WITH STRATEGIC (MARKET) PLANNING

Integrating the facility assessment with the internal market assessment during the strategic planning process brings a new dimension to this effort. For example, a review of facility strengths and weaknesses, along with potential facility and equipment capacity constraints and surpluses, may identify unforeseen opportunities for the organization to embark on new strategies with minimal risk. Alternately, the organization may decide early in the process to discard specific strategies that are deemed cost prohibitive.

Specifically, surplus space and equipment such as a vacant nursing unit or excess surgical capacity may provide quick and low-risk opportunities to launch a new program or grow an existing one with minimal capital investment. On the other hand, if new space must be constructed and equipped, the financial risk and the delayed timing could render a particular strategy less desirable.

If an organization is faced with a deteriorating physical plant that requires millions of dollars for infrastructure upgrading just to stay in business, then the strategic planning effort may be focused on revenue growth and financial viability.

BRIDGING THE GAP: UTILIZATION ANALYSES THAT ARE UNIQUE TO FACILITY PLANNING

Strategic plans for healthcare organizations vary in the degree to which specific strategies and actions are translated into quantified demand forecasts and tangible resource requirements such as facilities, equipment, and staff. A gap often exists between the action planning stage that concludes the strategic planning process and the input needed to commence the facility planning process. The translation of the organization's strategic planning initiatives and future service volumes into clinical service needs by location and corresponding space requirements is a critical aspect of facility master planning. Whether developed as part of the strategic planning process or as part of the facility planning process, identification of the following, at a minimum, is required:

- New programs and services that will require space or new facilities

- Future bed need by clinical service line, acuity, patient accommodation type, and location, including the development of "high-bed" and "low-bed" scenarios

- Ambulatory services strategy relative to projected demand, service delivery locations, and physician office needs

- Future ancillary workload projections (by location) for selected diagnostic and treatment services, with inpatient and outpatient breakdown

Strategies related to market penetration, physician recruitment, and customer satisfaction, along with other studies on the current status and future direction of key clinical service lines, should also be incorporated into the facility planning effort. In particular, detailed business plans for new or expanding clinical service lines provide a sound foundation for facility planning.

Even though analyses of current and historical inpatient utilization, bed need, and ancillary workload projections are commonly undertaken as part of the strategic planning process, a different perspective is required for facility planning.

HIGH-BED AND LOW-BED SCENARIOS

For facility planning purposes, projecting the need for an absolute number of beds at some future date is not nearly as important as identifying the range of beds required based on the most optimistic versus pessimistic view of future market conditions. This type of sensitivity analysis can help an organization understand the impact of forecasting inaccuracies. This is particularly important because decisions to expand or replace inpatient facilities start a chain reaction of events and involve a long-range commitment of dollars, staff time, and operational disruption.

Also, consider the fluctuation in demand for inpatient beds over the past several decades. With pressures from payers, both the rate of admission and length of stay dropped between 1980 and 2002, resulting in a rapid decline in inpatient utilization. Community hospitals took more than 167,000 inpatient beds out of service during this period. The downward trend in inpatient volumes began moderating in the mid-1990s as a backlash to managed care. In 1999, hospital patient days actually increased slightly after two decades of decline. Today, in a complete reversal of the trends of the 1990s, many hospitals are experiencing increased demand for inpatient care at a time when they have substantially reduced the resources allocated for inpatient care, are having difficulties accessing capital for facility renovation and expansion, and are faced with widespread staffing shortages (AHA and Lewin Group 2004). Over the next 25 years, the demand for inpatient beds in the United States is projected to increase by as much as 46 percent (an additional 238,000 beds) based on demographics alone with no change in use rates for both admissions and patient days (Solucient 2002).

Table 3.1 provides an example of a bed-need analysis that looks at the sensitivity of bed need to changes in the key variables of use rate, market share, length of stay, and occupancy rate. In this example, different scenarios were modeled based on varying market share, length of stay, and occupancy rate assumptions, with the use rate and projected service area population held constant. However, any one or all of

TABLE 3.1 COMPARING FUTURE BED-NEED SCENARIOS

	Current	Year 2010 Bed-Need Scenarios		
		Low Bed Need (Declining Market Share)	Medium Bed Need (Current Market Share)	High Bed Need (Increased Market Share)
Service area population	445,030	485,000	485,000	485,000
Use rate (admissions/1,000)	110.5	110.5	110.5	110.5
Hospital market share	27.6%	26.3%	27.6%	30.4%
Hospital admissions	13,573	14,095	14,792	16,292
Hospital length of stay	5.50	5.00	5.25	5.50
Hospital census	205	193	213	245
Bed need at				
90% occupancy		215	236	273
85% occupancy		227	250	289
80% occupancy		241	266	307
Current bed capacity	227	227	227	227
Bed surplus (+) or deficit (-)		+12 to -14	-9 to -39	-46 to -80

these variables can be modified to develop a realistic range of future bed need for a specific organization. The goal of this type of analysis is to evaluate the magnitude of renovation or construction necessary given the range of optimistic versus pessimistic scenarios. In Table 3.1, the low-bed scenario would have minimal impact. In the high-bed scenario, a major bed expansion would be required to accommodate two to three additional nursing units. In this particular example, some observations regarding the 2010 projections include the following:

- The 10 percent increase in population alone results in the need for an additional 50 beds at the 80 percent occupancy level.

- A 10 percent increase in *either* market share, use rate, or length of stay, has about the same effect on bed need (an additional 50 beds at 80 percent occupancy).

- Assuming a higher occupancy target of 90 percent versus 80 percent results in the need for approximately 13 percent fewer beds in all scenarios or the equivalent of one less nursing unit.

Historically, 80 percent occupancy was used as a target for acute medical and surgical nursing units. However, organizations with only private patient rooms are reevaluating this target. Given the high cost of construction and planning uncertainties, many financial officers are willing to accept the risk of not accommodating all demand during peak periods in lieu of having vacant patient rooms during average census periods. Statistically, a hospital with all private patient rooms should be able to maintain a higher occupancy level than one with a large number of semiprivate or multiple-bed rooms. Targeting a higher occupancy level is not practical for an organization with a high percentage of semiprivate patient rooms.

Target occupancy rates for an individual nursing unit or service line are generally a function of the nature of arrivals (random versus predictable), risk of not accommodating peak demand (intensive care versus behavioral health), the size of the service or unit, and seasonal fluctuations in demand. This is why intensive care, obstetrics, and pediatrics units may be planned with much lower target occupancy rates, such as 65 percent to 70 percent, and behavioral health units may be planned with higher rates, such as 90 percent.

EVALUATING BED SCENARIOS WHEN THERE IS A DEFICIT OF PRIVATE ROOMS

If your facility was constructed with only private patient rooms, then you can skip to the next section. Otherwise, you will be challenged with planning a staged conversion of semiprivate patient rooms to privates over time. However, this may offer you additional flexibility that could offset forecasting inaccuracies. If the low-bed scenario plays out, then some of the existing semiprivate patient rooms could be used as single occupancy. On the other hand, if the high-bed scenario comes to fruition, then the organization would need to deploy more of the rooms as semiprivates during peak census periods.

Now let's look at the example for another organization in Figure 3.1, where the mix of private and semiprivate patient rooms comes into play. This figure displays the high-bed and low-bed scenarios projected in five-year increments, along with the organization's existing design capacity (equal mix of privates and semiprivates) and actual number of patient rooms. With a total of 232 rooms, regardless of whether some were originally designed to accommodate two patients, this hospital would essentially operate as an all-private facility when the average daily census is 232 or less.

High-Bed Scenario

This organization could accommodate the high-bed need through 2010 if it chose to accommodate the current proportion of patients in semi-private rooms during peak census periods. Beyond 2010, bed expansion would definitely be required in the high-bed scenario. Prior to that point in time, assuming that the high-bed scenario comes to fruition, possible bed expansion strategies might include the following:

- Conservative approach: Construct 70 additional private rooms, thus increasing the proportion of private patient rooms to 60 percent.

- Aggressive approach: Construct up to 148 additional private rooms, resulting in 100 percent of the total beds being in private rooms.

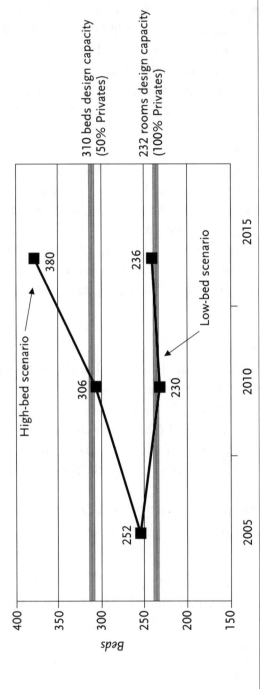

- A variation of the above approaches is possible, depending on the degree of confidence that the high-bed scenario will be achieved, the financial resources, and the desire to end up with 100 percent of the total beds being in private rooms.

Low-Bed Scenario

Because this facility was originally designed with a total of 232 patient rooms (154 privates and 78 semiprivates), each room in the low-bed scenario could essentially be used for single occupancy, and no expansion would be necessary through 2015.

SAME-DAY-STAY PATIENTS AND OBSERVATION BEDS

The forecasting of beds that are used for observation, with a length of stay generally less than 24 hours, also varies from one organization to the next. Nursing staff will often take issue with bed forecasts that fail to account for this growing group of patients that typically occupy inpatient beds. Although it is becoming more common for healthcare organizations to record these patients on daily census reports, most traditional bed-need methodologies are not designed to accommodate this group of patients. At a minimum, the current daily number of observation and same-day patients occupying an inpatient bed (but not counted in the midnight census) should be estimated based on central data sources or by conducting periodic data sampling unit by unit. With this data, the optimal setting for these patients should be identified—for example, inpatient bed, same-day medical procedure unit, or ED—and future assumptions regarding bed need by location (setting) can be confirmed.

LOCATION, LOCATION, LOCATION

The real estate investment mantra "location, location, location" is critical when assessing and projecting healthcare utilization data to be used for facility planning. Healthcare organizations collect data for many different purposes, most notably for financial accounting of revenue and costs. Data may also be used to evaluate operational efficiency and staff productivity. For facility planning purposes however, utilization data by location are most critical and often difficult to ascertain from forecasts of inpatient and ancillary service demand that are generated in a strategic plan.

Emergency visits and obstetrical deliveries (births) are often projected during the strategic planning process by applying use rates per 1,000 population and market share assumptions to forecast future (market-based) demand. However, the rigor of forecasting other ancillary workloads is often insufficient. Forecasts for major services—such as surgical cases; endoscopies; imaging procedures, including routine radiography and fluoroscopy, CT, MRI, positron emission testing (PET), nuclear medicine, and interventional; and invasive and noninvasive cardiology—are often developed by department or service-line managers (bottom-up approach). A typical methodology involves simply extending the historical trend forward to the designated future planning horizon. Inpatient and outpatient breakdowns may not even be delineated. The forecasting of less traditional service volumes such as hospital-based medical procedures, including transfusions, biopsies, IV therapy, and pulmonary function testing, is often even less scientific.

Procedure volumes gathered from central data sources do not typically designate the location where the procedures were performed, although department statistics are generally more detailed. Procedures performed at the point of care with portable equipment are often grouped with department-based inpatient or outpatient procedures. This is a particular problem with routine radiology, fluoroscopy, EKG, and ultrasound statistics, where procedures performed with portable equipment at the patient's bedside or in an outpatient clinic may represent a sizable proportion of the workload.

In general, ancillary workloads should be broken down into inpatient and outpatient components, and each should be projected separately. The inpatient component can be correlated to inpatient admissions by analyzing the historical ratio per admission and then applying a target ratio to the forecasted admissions. Projection of the outpatient component is far less scientific and should be qualitative based on market strategy, physician recruitment plans, pending reimbursement changes, and historical trends. Table 3.2 provides an example for forecasting surgery, CT, and MRI workloads.

Overly optimistic growth projections prepared by department or service-line managers should be challenged, particularly if they result in a decision to commit capital dollars to additional equipment, procedure rooms, and support space. Also, outpatient volumes that are erratic and show no discernable trend should be monitored. Knowledge of individual physicians and their status should also be incorporated

TABLE 3.2   EXAMPLE: PROJECTING ANCILLARY WORKLOADS

Med/Surg/ICU	2001	2002	2003	2004	2010	Comments
Admissions	26,578	27,165	28,423	29,375	41,000	Projected medical/surgical/ICU admissions

Surgery	2001	2002	2003	2004	2010	Comments
Open heart cases	1,288	1,303	1,334	1,296	1,296	Status quo assumed
Other IP cases	10,465	10,974	11,657	12,349	17,220	Calculated
IP cases/admission	0.39	0.40	0.41	0.42	0.42	Assumes current ratio will be maintained
OP cases	13,984	15,893	16,716	16,901	17,000	Will level off with off-site competition
% OP cases	54%	56%	56%	55%	48%	Calculated
Total Cases	25,737	28,170	29,707	30,546	35,516	

CT	2001	2002	2003	2004	2010	Comments
IP tests	9,350	10,220	11,519	12,169	16,810	Calculated
IP tests/admission	0.35	0.38	0.41	0.41	0.41	Assumes current ratio will be maintained
OP tests	17,410	21,187	22,788	23,980	32,130	Assumes growth of 5% a year
% OP tests	65%	67%	66%	66%	66%	Calculated
Total Tests	26,760	31,407	34,307	36,149	48,940	

MRI	2001	2002	2003	2004	2010	Comments
IP tests	2,107	2,256	2,294	2,456	3,280	Calculated
IP tests/admission	0.08	0.08	0.08	0.08	0.08	Assumes current ratio will be maintained
OP tests	5,910	5,822	6,005	6,320	7,120	Assumes growth of 2% per year
% OP tests	74%	72%	72%	72%	68%	Calculated
Total Tests	8,017	8,078	8,299	8,776	10,400	

into the projection of outpatient volumes. Examples may include the following:

- Surgeons who lack commitment to the organization and alternate between hospital-based and outpatient surgery facilities year to year or who are planning to invest in their own freestanding ambulatory surgery center;

- Cardiologists who alternate between competing organizations depending on which facility has the latest technology; and

- Physicians whose interest in performing specific procedures at the hospital-based facility, versus in their own offices, fluctuates depending on reimbursement and regulatory issues such as x-ray, endoscopy, ultrasound, and chemotherapy.

Highly productive physicians or surgeons who are close to retirement may also have a significant impact on future workload projections. Alternately, physician recruitment plans that could result in substantial workload growth should be factored into future workload forecasts. Unfortunately, I have seen many examples around the country where a physician specialist demanded new equipment and space from a trusting hospital administrator and then skipped across town to the competing hospital once the first hospital's new facilities opened.

PLANNING CENTERS OF EXCELLENCE

In the special situation where an organization is planning to realign and collocate specific treatments and procedures by service line, identifying and quantifying the specific workloads that will occur in the new center may be challenging. Caution should be exercised so that projected workloads are not double-counted, resulting in the planning of capacity at both a new specialty center and an existing hospital-based department or freestanding diagnostic facility.

LINKING THE CAPACITY ASSESSMENT TO FORECASTS OF FUTURE DEMAND

Incorporating the capacity assessment described in Chapter 5 into the workload forecasting effort is important. In the capacity assessment, the current capacity of each major clinical service is identified based on the current number of procedure rooms, the equipment and technology, and the specific operational characteristics; then the optimal capacity that could be achieved through operational changes, such as extended hours of operation, new equipment, and procedural changes, is defined. With this knowledge in hand, the workload forecasting activity can be focused on those services that are presently at or near capacity relative to projected future workload volumes.

For example, it may be determined that an existing surgery suite, where 70 percent of the cases are ambulatory, is averaging 750 annual cases per OR (three cases per day, 250 days per year), which is very low utilization. If weekday hours were extended such that one more case were added each day, the existing number of operating rooms could accommodate a 33 percent increase in workload. In this case, future workload forecasts would not need to be scrutinized unless explosive growth (beyond 33 percent) is anticipated. As another example, if an older CT unit, which accommodates 12 to 16 patients in an eight-hour shift, is replaced with a high-speed model that can accommodate 16 to 22 patients per shift, a 35 percent increase in workload could be achieved without facility expansion. If the same imaging suite were also able to staff and schedule patients for six hours on Saturdays, future growth of over 50 percent could be accommodated. With this kind of operational flexibility, little time needs to be spent debating the accuracy of forecasts from a facility planning perspective.

THE APPROPRIATE PLANNING HORIZON FOR FACILITY PLANNING

Much debate often takes place regarding appropriate planning horizons. Population-based forecasts of inpatient admissions, births, or ED visits must correspond with the planning horizons of the available population projections and will only be as accurate as the population forecasts on which they are based. At the same time, new healthcare facilities built today must meet the needs of patients for many decades beyond the standard five-year to ten-year strategic planning horizon. A prudent approach is to first understand the current and optimal capacity of existing equipment, procedure rooms, and support space and then to focus on those services where capacity is an issue. Finally, as discussed in Chapter 11, the planning of flexible, multiuse, or adaptable facilities can cost-effectively offset inaccuracies in workload forecasting. Unless a new or replacement healthcare facility is being planned, most healthcare organizations will translate their facility development strategies into immediate (within two years), short-term (within two to five years), and long-range (beyond five years) projects, as described in Chapter 7. This is necessary because of the length of the planning, design, and construction cycle; capital funding; and staff energy required to execute the facility master plan.

REFERENCES

American Hospital Association (AHA) and Lewin Group. 2004. *TrendWatch Chartbook 2004: Trends Affecting Hospitals and Health Systems.* Chicago: American Hospital Association.

Solucient. 2002. "National and Local Impact of Long-term Demographic Change on Inpatient Acute Care." Report. Evanston, IL: Solucient.

Zuckerman, A. 1998. *Healthcare Strategic Planning: Approaches for the 21st Century.* Chicago: Health Administration Press.

CHAPTER FOUR

Coordinating Operations Improvement Initiatives and Planned Technology Investments with Facility Planning

T O OPTIMIZE YOUR capital investments, facility planning should be integrated with institutionwide and service-line-specific operations improvement initiatives and also coordinated with planned information technology (IT) investments. This provides an opportunity for facility reconfiguration or expansion to potentially improve operational efficiency, enhance customer service, and provide future operational flexibility. Coordinating an organization's IT strategic planning efforts with long-range facility planning may offer new opportunities to unbundle current space and may improve the accuracy of the capital budgeting process. For example, assumptions regarding future capital outlays for computer hardware should be coordinated with long-range strategies regarding the functional use and future status of specific buildings or facility components, such as a change in functional use or demolition.

INSTITUTIONWIDE OPERATIONS IMPROVEMENT INITIATIVES

The objective of most of the operations reengineering efforts in which I was involved in the mid-1990s was to reduce the number of hospital departments and increase the span of control—for example, increasing the number of subordinates per manager or supervisor. Many departments were operating more or less autonomously, focused on their own bottom lines. From my experience, consolidation of traditional hospital departments through operations reengineering has been shown to do the following:

- improve both the continuity and quality of care with a more integrated provider team;

- enhance productivity through the cross-training of staff;

- enhance customer service and facilitate wayfinding with one-stop shopping; and

- generally provide more efficient use of staff, equipment, and space.

The ongoing movement toward patient-centered care responds to the need to redesign the patient-care delivery system such that the hospital resources and personnel are organized around the patient rather than around specialized departments. The current trend toward decentralization of many modalities to the point of care—for example, laboratory testing, imaging, and admitting—further challenges rigid departmental boundaries, organizational structures, and job descriptions.

What does this have to do with the facility planning process? In the traditional facility planning approach, the facility planner or programmer solicits input from individual department managers and their staff, which often results in the replication of existing, inefficient organizational structures and operational systems at a time when there is a tremendous opportunity to use facility reconfiguration as the impetus to affect operational change. Department leadership may be unaware of best practices occurring elsewhere, or they may be reluctant to challenge the status quo. Multidisciplinary task forces, focused on specific patient processes, may help department managers to think outside of the box. However, strong administrative leadership and participation is needed if organization structures are to be altered or if job descriptions are to be revised. Some organizations may not have the resources (or the energy) to embark on significant operations restructuring during predesign planning. Regardless, planning and designing selected staff workstations and procedure rooms contiguous with each other, such that staff from different departments work side by side, may eventually facilitate more formal operations reorganization and cross-training of staff.

COMMON INSTITUTIONWIDE SYSTEMS AND RELATED TECHNOLOGY

An understanding of common institutionwide operational systems, processes, and related technology in current use is critical to a successful facility planning effort. Specifically, current operational problems, priorities, and operations improvement opportunities should be identified related to the following:

- Customer expectations

- Departments exhibiting operational problems, particularly relating to multiple-site or divided operations

- Effectiveness of common institutionwide systems and related technology that affect resource utilization, such as staffing, equipment, and space, including

  - Wayfinding and orientation, outpatient registration, scheduling, and test result reporting to referring physicians
  - Inpatient admitting, discharge, billing, and collections
  - Health information management (medical records)
  - Patient transportation
  - Materials and supply chain management

- Departments perceived as having major facility deficiencies with regard to inappropriate space allocation and functional relationships, which affect operational efficiency

- Equipment or technology constraints and anticipated improvements

- Recent developments, trends, and operations improvement initiatives that will significantly affect facility needs, such as e-health initiatives and electronic archiving

Once documented, assumptions regarding future changes can then be incorporated into the facility planning process.

CLINICAL SERVICE-LINE OPERATIONS IMPROVEMENT INITIATIVES

Operations improvement initiatives for specific clinical service lines such as emergency, surgery, or imaging should also be reviewed and appropriate operational assumptions incorporated into assessments of capacity and workload throughput as part of the facility planning process. If successfully implemented, such operational improvements may have a dramatic effect on the need for exam and treatment spaces, overall space, and ultimately construction costs. Table 4.1 illustrates the relationship between ED performance, as measured by treatment space turnaround time, and the number of annual visits that can be accommodated in each treatment space.

THE DIGITAL HOSPITAL

The digital transformation of America's 5,000 hospitals is underway. On the administrative side, electronic claims are universal, purchasing is automated, and communications are mostly by e-mail. On the clinical side, medical records are becoming computerized, images are being stored using picture archiving and communication systems (PACS), decision support software is determining nursing care plans, and computerized physician order entry (CPOE) is becoming the standard of care. Handheld personal digital assistants (PDAs), high-speed communication networks, and wireless technology are widely available. Pocket radio phones are replacing the use of overhead pagers that once prompted care providers to find wall telephones. Barcoding is being used to reduce medical errors, track supply inventories, capture patient supply charges, and reduce materials management labor costs (Coile 2003).

TABLE 4.1   RELATIONSHIP BETWEEN ED PERFORMANCE AND CAPACITY

Emergency Department Performance	Average Treatment Space Turnaround Time (Minutes)	Average Annual Visits per Treatment Space
Poor	180	1,100 to 1,200
Average	150	1,300 to 1,600
Best	120	1,700 to 1,900

Source: Hayward, C. 2005. *SpaceMed—A Space Planning Guide for Healthcare Facilities.* Ann Arbor, MI: Hayward & Associates, LLC. [Online information; retrieved 7/21/05.] www.space-med.com.

The lynchpin of the digital hospital, however, is the electronic medical record (EMR), and the nation's "100 most wired" hospitals are making significant progress in automating its key components. According to a survey by *Hospital and Health Networks* (2004), 90 percent reported online access to the patient's current medical record, with 87 percent able to access the patient's medical history and 69 percent able to access nurses' notes online. However, this transition has not occurred as quickly as anticipated a decade ago. According to *Futurescan 2003*, a survey of 420 healthcare CEOs, executives, strategists, marketers, and communicators, only 55 percent agreed that EMRs in hospitals will become the standard of practice in the next two to five years (Coile 2003).

Rapid advances in information and telecommunication technologies are creating new staff positions and revised job descriptions, as well as altering historical perceptions about necessary physical proximities and functional relationships between departments. Many traditional health and financial data management functions are being consolidated—for example, medical records, quality assurance, risk management, infection control, finance, data processing, and telecommunications—as multiple types of data can be obtained expeditiously from common databases. As a result, many staff that once required face-to-face contact with patients and visitors no longer need to occupy prime space on the main floor of an acute care hospital and can be relocated to any place with a phone and Internet access.

Imagine a scenario where every member of the healthcare administrative staff is assigned a mobile computing device such as a laptop computer, PDA, or cellular phone in lieu of an office, desk, file cabinets, bookshelves, and hard-wired computer and phone. Whether the staff member is an administrator, nurse manager, financial analyst, surgery scheduler, IT programmer, or a registration clerk, he or she either works from home, where management objectives can be quantified; works in a central administrative office suite (or building) in an assigned office or cubicle; or works directly at the point of care, or point of service, to facilitate the needs of the organization's patients and other customers.

Using wireless technology, all staff can access the institution's secure intranet and external Internet to input, retrieve, review, analyze, and store all data and information required to fulfill the requirements of their specific role within the organization. In this paperless environment, all day-to-day communication occurs electronically via e-mail or voice mail, and routine management reports and information such as time sheets, budgets, and personnel assessments are all created, transmitted, and stored electronically. This scenario seems somewhat futuristic when envisioned for the healthcare industry, even though this is the standard mode of operation today for many other industries.

IMPACT OF E-HEALTH

The Healthcare Information and Management Systems Society (HIMSS 2003) defines e-health as "The application of the Internet and other related technologies in the healthcare industry to improve the access, efficiency, effectiveness, and quality of clinical and business processes utilized by healthcare organizations, practitioners, patients, and consumers to improve the health status of patients." E-health is changing the way information is collected, stored, and disseminated, and the medical center of today is being redefined as healthcare organizations change the way that they interact with patients and families, physicians, employees, payers, vendors, and other institutional partners. Some examples of changing interactions and processes include the following:

- *Patient and family interaction.* The hospital's web site is being used as the initial point of contact for the patient and his or her family prior to arrival. Face-to-face preadmission and registration; scheduling; financial counseling; case and disease management; patient education and research; and family, clergy, and community communications are being supplemented (and often replaced) by Internet communications.

- *Physician interaction.* Medical staff credentialing, continuing education, clinical research and clinical trials, results reporting, and referrals and consultations are done online; telemedicine allows remote diagnostics and therapeutics with efficient clinical data transmission and image management.

- *Employee interaction.* Recruiting, benefits enrollment and administration, in-service education, work life, and legal issues can all be accommodated online using a secure intranet.

- *Payer interaction.* All data for claims processing, benefits eligibility, clinical outcomes, and contracting can be exchanged electronically in a standardized format and over a secure network.

- *Vendor and supplier interaction.* Electronic data interchange (EDI), universal product codes, barcoding, and radio frequency identification (RFID) systems result in new and different processes, workflow, and facility needs.

The creation of a paperless healthcare environment that exploits Internet, mobile, and wireless technologies is having a revolutionary impact on the need for physical proximity between departments and functional areas that was deemed necessary in the past. Thus, many of the traditional facility planning principles that were based on the need for departments to share paper, equipment, and patients are no longer relevant. This new, virtual-workplace phenomenon allows large numbers of individuals or groups to work collaboratively with the assistance of modern, computer-based communications technologies, and it involves all employees who do not require direct face-to-face interaction with their customers. In addition, the use of the Internet to enhance the organization's image and brand identity, as well as its uses for promotion, advertising, and community awareness, is supplementing one of the traditional roles of the bricks and mortar.

In addition to communication technologies, other new technologies are beginning to influence medical practice and create new possibilities for patient diagnosis and treatment. The need for less space in large centralized departments often results as equipment is miniaturized, made more mobile, and decentralized to the point of care. Less space will also be needed for staff who may telecommute and for on-site hard-copy record storage.

CONSIDERING NEW OPERATIONAL AND FACILITY CONFIGURATION MODELS

By embarking on institutionwide operations reengineering, healthcare organizations have been challenging traditional, inefficient organizational structures and operational systems over the past several decades. However, some of the benefits of reengineering can only be achieved though physical facility reconfiguration. For example, the physical reorganization and consolidation of similar functions enhance operational efficiency, create opportunities for cross-training of staff, and reduce the number of managers and supervisors. This may result in a reduction in space need, because smaller staffs require fewer offices and workstations, and quicker throughput lessens the need for expensive procedure rooms and large patient and visitor waiting areas.

New operational models are emerging that not only enhance operational efficiency and optimize the use of scarce resources, such as staff, equipment, and space, but also improve customer service and promote future flexibility. All of these require some degree of facility reconfiguration and should be considered when major facility expansion or replacement for any of these services is being considered.

Some of the new operational models in which I have been involved are listed and described below:

- Developing a customer service center

- Consolidating express testing services

- Collocating specialty imaging and diagnostic services

- Rethinking interventional services

- Developing a medical procedure unit

- Rethinking the surgery center

- Rethinking the traditional intensive care unit (ICU)

- Planning for the laboratory of the future

- Planning the pharmacy of the future

- Creating a generic administrative office suite

- Unbundling building support services

These new concepts seldom emerge when a traditional facility planning process is deployed—for example, if the process is led by a designer or architect with input from department "silos." Implementation of these concepts requires an enlightened leadership team that is willing to challenge the status quo.

Developing a Customer Service Center
In the traditional healthcare facility, multiple departments and staff are commonly involved in customer intake, access, and processing activities such as the following:

- Reception, information dissemination, and wayfinding or orientation are often provided by volunteers.

- Inpatient admitting, outpatient registration, coordination of multiple appointments, and scheduling of follow-up appointments are often performed by one or more departments, such as the admitting department, central outpatient registration, or separate scheduling systems within individual diagnostic/treatment departments.

- Cashiering, insurance verification, billing, and financial counseling are performed by the finance department.

- Patient amenities may be dispersed with insufficient volume at any given location to warrant fixed staffing or facility upgrading.

This typically results in fragmented customer service and complicates wayfinding. Although many of these departments are located on the first floor of the facility, only a few staff in each department actually have face-to-face interaction with visitors, patients, and their families. The question is, How can an organization better utilize its staff and its space to both enhance operational efficiency and improve customer service?

With the continuing focus on patient-centered care and the emergence of multihospital systems, IT, and reengineering techniques, the trend is to consolidate customer intake, processing, and support services into a single operational unit. Such units are often referred to as a *customer service center, patient service center, access services,* or a similar designation. I prefer the term "customer," because it can refer to visitors, family members, employers, payers, physicians, staff, and vendors in addition to the patient who is scheduled for an interview, examination, procedure, or admission.

The customer service center is the primary patient and visitor intake, processing, and communication area for a healthcare facility or campus and also includes centralized patient and visitor amenities as shown in Figure 4.1. The customer service center should be located directly inside the primary entrance to the healthcare complex to serve as the initial access point for visitors and most scheduled patients. This area can also function as a "home base" for family members and visitors who are spending increased time at the facility as more treatments and procedures are performed on a same-day basis. Functional components of the customer service center typically include the following:

- *Central reception/intake and communication area,* including the entrance vestibule, initial reception and communication station for dissemination of information and orientation, family and visitor lounge, discharge lounge, public toilets, phones, automated teller machine (ATM), Internet kiosk, and other amenities for patients and visitors

FIGURE 4.1 CUSTOMER SERVICE CENTER CONCEPT

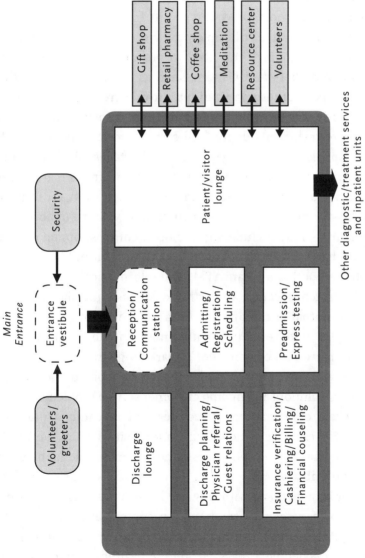

Source: Hayward, C. 2005. *SpaceMed—A Space Planning Guide for Healthcare Facilities.* Ann Arbor, MI: Hayward & Associates, LLC. [Online information; retrieved 7/21/05.] www.space-med.com.

- *Patient processing and access services*, including admitting, registration, insurance verification, scheduling, cashiering, billing, financial counseling, discharge planning, physician referral, patient and guest relations, and security

- *Other optional services*, such as a patient library/resource center, an outpatient or retail pharmacy, coffee shop, gift shop, spiritual or pastoral care, and support space for volunteers

Patients and visitors are spending longer time periods at acute care hospitals as more procedures shift from an inpatient stay to a same-day stay with a multiple-hour recovery period. Healthcare organizations recognize the need to provide appropriate amenities for family members and visitors, such as a comfortable family and visitor lounge. Some organizations provide free health screenings, utilize wall space for ongoing art exhibits, provide entertainment, and offer refreshments using food carts in or near the lounge. With many hospitals experiencing severe bed shortages, discharge lounges are becoming increasingly popular as a way to free inpatient rooms for the next patient while the discharged patient waits for transportation to his or her home. Other patient and visitor support services and amenities may include a gift shop, a coffee shop, an outpatient or retail pharmacy, a chapel or meditation room, public toilet facilities, phone booths, and an ATM. Durable medical equipment—for example, crutches, canes, and orthotic devices—may be dispensed as part of an outpatient pharmacy. Creating a welcoming and healing environment with enhanced amenities should be considered a necessary part of an organization's marketing strategy.

The healthcare industry is beginning to look to the hospitality industry for solutions to ongoing customer service problems that result from archaic organizational structures and inadequate information systems. For example, when a customer visits a hotel, he or she is greeted by a central reception desk and a comfortable lobby immediately upon entry. At this central reception desk, the customer can receive, or be networked with, any needed services; customers can register, pay bills, receive or send faxes, get information and directions, make a special request regarding housekeeping services, arrange transportation, or schedule a massage. Yet the healthcare industry requires that its customers visit multiple locations and interact with multiple staff and fragmented systems, assuming that the customer can first determine the appropriate access point for their needed service. The customer service center attempts to replicate the main reception desk typically found in an upscale hotel by using the same hub-and-spoke concept.

Consolidating Express Testing Services

Healthcare organizations are also consolidating high-volume, quick-turnaround diagnostic services into an express testing center that is often collocated with the customer service center to provide one-stop shopping. These services may include routine blood and urine collection, EKGs, chest x-rays, simple bone x-rays, and preadmission or presurgery consultation. For many acute care hospitals, a significant portion of their outpatient activity involves these routine services, yet patients are often expected to travel to multiple department locations throughout the hospital complex.

In both of these models, all staff work together as a team to provide quality care in an expedient manner. The staff are often cross-trained and report organizationally to a single supervisor rather than to multiple department managers. Patient satisfaction generally improves as wayfinding is simplified, patient throughput is expedited, waiting times are decreased, and continuity of care is improved, thus reducing operational costs. Less space is needed on the first floor (prime real estate) and staff that is not directly involved in face-to-face customer contact are relocated.

Some organizations may choose to locate an *express testing center* adjacent to the lobby of a major medical office building or ambulatory care center to enhance convenience for patients who are simultaneously visiting a physician or to provide more convenient parking and access. However, the key to successful implementation of this concept is to have sufficient utilization (high volumes) so as not to duplicate resources unnecessarily.

Collocating Specialty Imaging and Diagnostic Services

In an era of continued pressures to reduce costs, the planning of imaging services is challenging, because many hospitals have been historically engaged in an arms race to acquire the newest, and usually most expensive, technology. The shortage of radiology technologists, acquisition cost of new equipment, inadequate reimbursement (particularly where cost effectiveness has not yet been proven), and the turf wars between radiologists and other specialties are all current issues. Figure 4.2 illustrates the cost of acquiring new technology in today's environment.

With the convergence of specialty imaging technologies and modalities, as well as the ability to cost effectively provide routine imaging at the point of care, traditional departmental boundaries (and physical organization of space) are being challenged. Examples of converging specialty imaging modalities include the new hybrid imaging devices that combine PET and CT and PET and MRI. By combining the structural and functional information in a single scan, these equipment units allow the images to be fused, providing clinicians much more information than either scan would provide alone. At the same time, the cost of acquiring and maintaining portable imaging devices at the patient bedside or in outpatient clinics is decreasing.

The reality is that regardless of the specific imaging modality, all of these services use essentially the same types of space, including the following:

- Patient reception/registration and family waiting space

- Patient preparation space, such as gowning and injections

- Exam and consultation rooms

- Small procedures rooms to accommodate portable equipment such as ultrasound and EKG

- Large procedure rooms with fixed equipment that require more complicated design features, such as CT, MRI, PET, and interventional procedures

- Optional patient recovery space

- Procedure room support space such as storage and equipment cleaning

- Staff work space, such as reading/interpretation and administrative work

FIGURE 4.2 COST OF ACQUIRING NEW TECHNOLOGY

Traditional Technology		Contemporary Technology		Next-Round Technology
x-ray machine	⟶	CT scanner	⟶	CT functional imaging with PET
$175,000		$1,000,000		$2,300,000
Open-surgery instrument set	⟶	Laparoscopic surgery set	⟶	Robotic surgical device
$10,000		$15,000		$1,000,000
Cardiac balloon catheter	⟶	Stent	⟶	Treated stent
$500		$2,300		$5,000
Scalpel	⟶	Electrocautery	⟶	Harmonic scalpel
$20		$12,000		$30,000

Source: Cited with permission from the University HealthSystem Consortium.

Because of this, many healthcare organizations are collocating and consolidating traditional diagnostic and therapeutic departments to optimize the short-term sharing of resources and long-term flexibility. A single patient destination, such as a diagnostic center, may be provided to facilitate patient wayfinding. Patient intake and reception, family waiting, and preparation and recovery space may be shared and procedure rooms designed to flexibly accommodate changing equipment over time. Staff, particularly clerical and support staff, are also being cross-trained to the extent possible. Even though high-volume services may be able to justify the allocation of dedicated support staff and space, the collocation of procedure rooms and recovery space provides enhanced future flexibility that cannot be achieved with disparate service locations.

Depending on workload volumes and physical limitations, a small facility may have a single diagnostic center, and a large facility may continue to provide some specialization such as a diagnostic center as well as a separate specialty imaging center that may include MRI and PET. Because of rapidly changing technology, future flexibility is ensured by providing generic, multipurpose procedure rooms (and often equipment) where appropriate. With the focus on customer service as well as the sharing of staff and space (and in some cases, equipment), support staff should be cross-trained where applicable and should report to a limited number of supervisors and a single manager.

As the speed of new imaging devices increases—for example, a multislice CT scanner takes only six minutes per procedure—the amount of time needed to move the patient into and out of the room does not change, thus putting increased emphasis on the supporting processes and space to gain improvements in productivity to offset the increased equipment expense.

Rethinking Interventional Services

Healthcare organizations are also increasingly planning a single interventional suite, often contiguous with the surgery suite that can be shared by interventional radiologists and cardiologists in lieu of planning a separate catheterization laboratories and angiography rooms in the radiology department. This model provides increased future flexibility as clinical programs and medical staff change over time, which may result in a reduction in the number of total procedure rooms that need to be upgraded or constructed. It also minimizes the amount of space needed for patient reception and intake, family waiting, and patient preparation and recovery. The greatest challenge to this model involves the turf issues between the interventional radiologists and cardiologists and the promotion of the cardiology center of excellence.

Developing a Medical Procedure Unit

Historically, same-day medical procedures have been scattered throughout the hospital or ambulatory care facility, with redundant patient reception and waiting, preparation, recovery, instrument processing, and treatment spaces. Often, locations were selected to optimize historical reimbursement mechanisms. Some healthcare organizations are consolidating various same-day medical procedures in an area that functions as the equivalent of the same-day surgery center. The destination is often referred to as a *medical procedure unit*. Medical procedures may include endoscopies, bronchoscopies, and similar procedures as well as IV therapy, blood transfusions, infusions, para/thoracentesis, liver biopsies, and the preparation and recovery of patients undergoing various imaging procedures. This concept, as with others discussed in this chapter, requires new job descriptions and new space. The space generally includes a patient reception/intake and family waiting area, several procedure spaces (enclosed rooms and open or partially enclosed treatment bays), patient preparation and recovery cubicles, and related support space. Optimal flexibility can be achieved by collocating the medical procedure unit's recovery bays with one or more ED treatment "pods" such that a block or module of treatment and recovery bays can be cross-utilized to meet peaks and valleys of demand. The collocation of the medical procedure unit treatment and recovery bays with the same-day surgery recovery area can achieve the same flexibility.

Rethinking the Surgery Center

During the 1980s, many surgical procedures traditionally performed on an inpatient basis shifted to outpatient settings. These were relatively minor procedures that required a short recovery or observation period prior to discharge. Today, some of these procedures are performed in physician offices. The advent of minimally invasive surgical techniques in the 1990s introduced the second wave of surgical procedures from inpatient to outpatient settings. These more complex procedures, such as gallbladder removal, typically require a more lengthy recovery prior to discharge.

Although freestanding ambulatory surgery centers could easily accommodate the first wave of outpatient procedures, accommodating this second wave of minimally invasive procedures is more difficult for two reasons. First, minimally invasive surgical equipment is expensive and requires more highly trained staff, making duplication in multiple settings costly unless volumes are high. Second, most freestanding surgery centers are not designed to accommodate extended patient recovery periods, such as 12 or more hours, and lack the necessary support systems for extended hours of operation, such as dietary support, off-shift staffing, and security. The growing population of same-day-stay patients within the traditional acute care hospital requires efficient outpatient registration and processing systems, enhanced outpatient preparation and recovery space, and expanded family waiting areas and other amenities.

To respond to cost-containment pressures driven by a managed care environment and declining reimbursement, healthcare organizations are focusing on reducing operational costs. Physicians are focused on using their time as efficiently as possible. Consequently, many of the freestanding ambulatory surgery centers created in the 1980s to emphasize patient convenience are being consolidated with inpatient surgery suites to avoid unnecessary duplication of expensive equipment, to reduce physician travel time between multiple sites, and to eliminate other physician inconveniences such as variability of staffing and instrumentation. From my experience, freestanding ambulatory surgery suites are successful if volume is adequate to fully utilize them, if marketing opportunities to capture incremental revenue exist, if workload volumes can justify the duplication of resources, or if a freestanding facility is a requirement for legal or financial reasons.

From my experience, outpatient, short-stay, and same-day admit procedures may account for over 70 percent of a community hospital's surgical workload, causing those organizations to rethink the definition of ambulatory surgery. In the past two decades, physically separating inpatient and outpatient surgery has garnered some interest. Today, if space is inadequate to provide a single surgery suite, then innovative organizations are creating separate tertiary surgery suites, such as cardiac and neurosurgery, which can benefit from an adjacency with an ICU. All remaining outpatient and short-stay surgery, regardless of the length of recovery, is combined. Most same-day or short-stay surgery utilizes the same processes and resources regardless of whether the patient's recovery is two hours, six hours, or 30 hours. Regardless of the length of stay, these patients all arrive as an outpatient on the same day as their procedure.

Rethinking the Traditional ICU

I have observed that many hospitals feel that they never have enough intensive care beds and are constantly pressured to either expand existing units or create new units. Historically, ICUs have provided intensive observation and treatment of patients in unstable condition. Because of the high-tech requirements and highly skilled staff, these units are expensive to build and operate. Insufficient intensive care beds also affect the ED, as high-acuity patients waiting to be admitted clog the ED when the ICUs are full.

ICU beds proliferated in the era of cost-based reimbursement despite a lack of data supporting the effectiveness of aggregating patients in a specially configured unit. I have reviewed a number of patient acuity studies that have shown that many ICU patients are either too ill or too well to benefit from ICUs. At the same time, some healthcare organizations have built additional ICUs that they were unable to staff as a result of recruiting difficulties in a tight job market.

Many healthcare organizations are redesigning ICUs to better monitor and care for patients and are hiring specialists, known as *intensivists*, and are improving nurse-staffing ratios. Remote patient management of critically ill patients is being successfully implemented in a number of hospitals around the United States in response to shortages of nurses and intensivists, as well as pressures to improve the quality of care and patient outcomes. Remote, or virtual, ICU monitoring centers can monitor multiple ICUs at once from a remote location with real-time "telepresence," including the review of clinical documentation and medical images, the monitoring of vital signs, and the use of digital stethoscopes and high-quality video cameras. Use of a remote patient management system—for example, the eICU® solution patented by VISICU—allows scarce nursing and physician-intensivist staff to be more effectively leveraged 24/7 and can provide quicker identification of problems, faster intervention, improved outcomes, and lower operational costs. This system also provides rural hospitals with improved access to intensive care resources.

With changing reimbursement, a shortage of specially trained personnel, advances in technology, and limited access to capital dollars for facility renovation or expansion, I have found that hospitals are looking for alternatives to traditional ICUs. Some options may include the following:

- *Acuity-adaptable patient rooms* allow for staffing and equipment to be more readily adjusted to meet the needs of patients, thereby eliminating unnecessary transfers, potential overstaffing, and excessive treatment based on ICU protocols. Instead, critically ill patients, regardless of their location within the hospital, would be monitored remotely using the eICU concept.

- *Chest pain centers*, typically located in or proximate to the ED, can provide extended observation and evaluation of patients complaining of chest pain and can eliminate unnecessary admissions to a cardiac ICU.

- *Chronic ventilator units* provide care for ventilator-dependent patients who have been traditionally cared for in expensive ICUs because of the absence of alternative facilities.

- *Day recovery centers* are alternatives to cardiac ICUs for patients requiring cardiac monitoring for 12 to 24 hours following invasive cardiac procedures.

- *Extended recovery room hours* accommodate surgical patients who require 12 to 24 hours of intensive, post-operative observation prior to being transferred to general care units or being discharged.

Planning for the Laboratory of the Future

In the past, laboratory operations were organized by discipline, and the facilities were subdivided into numerous small rooms to reflect this organization. With the advent of automated technology, robotics, and the demand for rapid turnaround times by clinicians, clinical laboratories are being functionally reconfigured by testing methodology and turnaround time. Laboratory managers who seek to reorganize clinical testing along these lines often find that the physical facility is a barrier to more efficient operations. Instead of compartmentalized space, contemporary laboratories need open, flexible space that easily accommodates new technology, allows staff to freely work among many areas, and can be eventually converted to a totally automated laboratory.

Over the next several years, patients and physicians will view point-of-care testing for blood analysis as a standard of care, with the growing focus on reducing medical errors, eliminating process inefficiencies, and expediting care delivery. Approximately 30 percent to 50 percent of laboratory testing will occur at the point of care, either at the patient's bedside, ED, surgical suite, physician's office, or other ambulatory care setting. As shown in the example in Figure 4.3, the turnaround time between traditional laboratory testing in a central department and point-of-care testing is substantial.

In the future, the testing location and the scope of services provided will be determined by the turnaround time required. At a minimum,

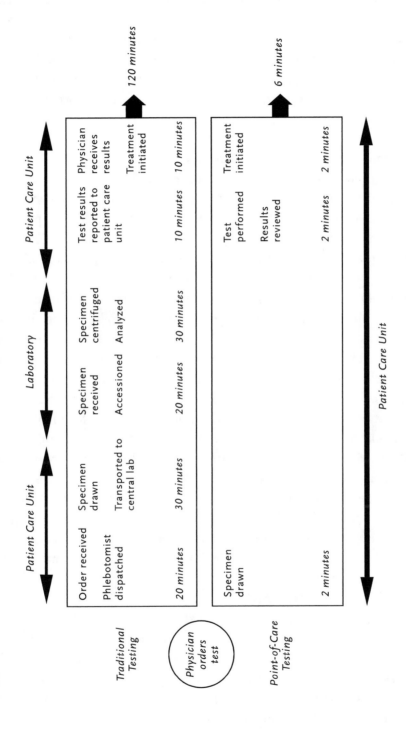

Source: Hayward, C. 2005. SpaceMed—A Space Planning Guide for Healthcare Facilities. Ann Arbor, MI: Hayward & Associates, LLC. [Online information; retrieved 7/21/05.] www.space-med.com.

hospitals will have point-of-care laboratories at key sites and on-site rapid response laboratories to provide testing on specimens requiring less than a 24-hour turnaround time. Regional reference laboratories (providing testing on specimens with a turnaround time of greater than 24 hours) will be developed to take advantage of new technology or specialized expertise. Initially, reference work may be divided between facilities—for example, housing all microbiology at one hospital and all special chemistry at another—to fully utilize existing space, staff, and equipment.

Planning the Pharmacy of the Future

The type of space traditionally planned within the central pharmacy will change because of new technologies that include barcodes and automated drug dispensing machines (ADDMs). In addition, pharmacist workstations in the central pharmacy and on the nursing units will need to be reconfigured to handle the electronic verification of medication orders rather than the receipt of hard copies of orders. Any manual processes for transporting the hard copies of physician orders to the pharmacist will no longer be needed—for example, human transport, fax machines, and pneumatic tube systems—resulting in significant space redesign. In addition, a number of tasks will no longer be necessary, such as pharmacist order entry from the hard copy, label generation, medication filling, medication checking, and delivery to nursing units as well as nurses searching for medications and administering them from a manual medication administration record. Space for these activities can be shifted to support new technology or can be eliminated as needed.

In the past, pharmacies depended on large, wheeled carts to deliver 24-hour supplies of scheduled medications and "as needed," or "prn," medications to the nursing units. The pharmacy technician and pharmacist traditionally used "fill lists" to fill and check the medication carts that demanded large amounts of floor space and a large work area within the central pharmacy. With the use of ADDMs, 24-hour cart exchanges will be greatly diminished. Space will still be required to select medications needed for replacement into the ADDMs, but because this process is no longer patient-name driven, cart size and fill areas may be reduced. The size and shape of IV rooms may also be reduced as some pharmacies commit to the use of outsourcing of total parenteral nutrition and other large volume parenterals. Improved inventory practices such as just-in-time delivery, multiday delivery, and direct delivery to ADDMs will reduce inventory storage requirements and will shift some of the current inventories to a central warehouse off site.

As many pharmacy distribution processes are automated, some pharmacist hours may be directed to more clinical duties. These clinical duties may reduce the need for space in the central (distribution) pharmacy and allow these clinical professionals to spend more time on the nursing units.

Creating a Generic Administrative Office Suite

The traditional healthcare facility has many departments involved in the administration and management of the organization in accordance with policies established by the governing board. Most of these central administrative services use generic office space with a mix of private offices, open or partially enclosed cubicles, and open workstations to accommodate different hierarchies of staff as dictated by the organizational structure and peak-shift staffing. Patient traffic to these areas is rare.

With the traditional organization of healthcare institutions into multiple, numerous departments, each with dedicated space and narrowly defined job descriptions, efficient space utilization was difficult to achieve. As many of these departments were forced to resize their staff in response to cost-containment pressures and changing skill requirements, vacant offices and workstations were scattered throughout the organization. At times, growing departments would need to compress multiple people into a single office, while shrinking departments had surplus space. Many departments also had dedicated conference rooms, which although infrequently used, were not available for use by other hospital services.

The trend toward the planning of generic administrative office suites, with a central reception and waiting area and groups of conference rooms, provides the most efficient space utilization and ensures that space is equitably allocated and distributed among the departments and services that need it at any given time. The intent is to assign offices and workstations according to the immediate need, allowing for the flexibility to reassign the space on a periodic basis as demand changes. This prevents staff from becoming overly "territorial" about their space. With more sophisticated information systems, space can still be charged to department or cost center budgets based on use and conference rooms or classrooms scheduled can centrally be based on demand.

Unbundling Building Support Services

Also referred to as "hotel services," building support services include materials management, central sterile processing, dietary services, and environmental and building maintenance services. Just as the clinical areas of the healthcare organization are undergoing operational reengineering to become more patient centered, building support services are changing to make services available on demand to meet patient needs. New operational concepts ensure the availability of supplies and equipment as needed, the delivery of dietary trays at the proper temperature when the patient is ready, and the completion of housekeeping and building maintenance services at the patient's convenience. Although a kitchen is one of the most expensive areas to build and equip within a medical center, most other building services require less expensive, industrial-type space. In most organizations, these functions can share a common administrative area and staff support facilities.

Because of the high cost of space built to acute care hospital standards, building support services are being reconfigured to use less (particularly less expensive) space. Just-in-time delivery and stockless materials management models place the burden of storage on the vendor, and the decentralization of other services to the point of care also reduces the amount of space needed in a large central department. Many of these services could appropriately be located adjacent to, or separate from, the acute care facility in a less expensive building (or service center) connected by a tunnel or an enclosed walkway. Multihospital healthcare systems are finding that it is less costly to support multiple hospital sites from a centralized service center that is remote from one or more hospital sites.

Unfortunately, many existing hospitals were originally designed to support a much larger number of inpatient beds than are currently staffed. With the shift to outpatient and same-day services that require less intensive building support services, many older facilities have a much larger chassis than currently needed. The typical older hospital was designed with building support services generally located in the basement or on a subgrade level. Many healthcare facilities today are plagued by a "rabbit's warren" of underground spaces that have received little upgrading or renovation since the time that the original facility was built. Any new healthcare facility being planned today should consider locating building support services in a separate, less costly, adjacent (or attached) building that does not have to be built to the more stringent inpatient building codes.

NOTE

1. For additional reference, see Hayward, C. 2005. *SpaceMed—A Space Planning Guide for Healthcare Facilities*. Ann Arbor, MI: Hayward & Associates, LLC. [Online information; retrieved 7/21/05.] www.space-med.com.

REFERENCES

Coile, R. C., Jr. 2003. *Futurescan 2003: A Forecast of Healthcare Trends 2003–2007*. Chicago: Society for Healthcare Strategy and Market Development, American Hospital Association.

Healthcare Management Information Systems Society (HIMSS). 2003. [Online press release; retrieved 7/21/05.] www.himss.org/pressroom.

Hospital and Health Networks. 2004. *Most Wired Hospitals and Benchmarking Study*. Chicago: American Hospital Association.

CHAPTER FIVE

Identifying Facility Needs and Establishing Priorities

WITH AN UNDERSTANDING of your current situation, future market strategy and projected demand, and potential operations improvement opportunities and technology investments, current and future facility needs can be identified and priorities established. The first step is to determine your space needs by location on a department (or service line) basis so that the magnitude of current and future space shortages can be known. Other facility deficiencies can then be identified, summarized, and prioritized. Key questions include the following:

- How well do we orient our customers as they arrive on the campus and circulate through our facilities?

- What is the workload capacity of our current facilities?

- Do we have enough space to support our current and projected number of licensed and staffed beds, procedure rooms, staff, and other required functions?

- Is our space organized and configured appropriately?

UNDERSTANDING THE SPACE PLANNING PROCESS

Space planning typically requires varying levels of detail at different points in the facility planning process. During the facility master planning stage, a broad-brush approach is used to assess the magnitude of current and future space shortages. Using each department's footprint, a comparison is made between the current space allocation, the current space need (based on current services, workload, equipment, staffing, etc.), and the future space need (based on program growth, new services, and anticipated operational and technology changes). The resulting preliminary space projections are used to develop facility reconfiguration options, site plans, and department block diagrams as part of the facility master plan. The planning horizon should correspond to the workload forecasts discussed in Chapter 3. For the purposes of facility master planning, the space requirements of individual departments are estimated in the aggregate DGSF, which differs from the detailed, room-by-room space programming in NSF as described in Chapter 8. Detailed, room-by-room space programming is generally undertaken after specific projects have been defined as an outcome of the facility master plan.

The approach to preliminary space planning depends on the organization's objectives, immediate issues, and corporate culture. The broad-brush approach is used to assess the overall scope of space deficiencies. Detailed, room-by-room space programming is not routinely performed at the facility master planning stage because it entails a tremendous amount of staff time and energy that is not appropriate for all departments, particularly those whose facilities are not an issue and whose status quo is assumed for the near future. In some cases, a more focused approach may be appropriate for one or more departments or service lines, and the detailed space programming process may be "fast-tracked" during the facility master planning process. Examples may include situations when there is a competitive threat that requires a shortened planning or design schedule, such as an ambulatory surgery center or cancer center joint venture with physicians; when code noncompliances must be rectified immediately; or when major pieces of equipment require urgent replacement. In these cases, a decision may be made to overlap the more detailed operational and space programming process for selected departments with the overview space planning assessment for all other departments during the facility master planning phase.

TOOLS AND TECHNIQUES

At the onset of the facility master planning process, a preliminary list of all nursing units, departments, and functional areas should be assembled that corresponds to the institution's formal organizational structure or cost-center listing. Specific tools and techniques are discussed below.

Focused Data Collection, Interviewing, and Surveying

Many facility planning consultants use standardized questionnaires to collect baseline data from department managers and medical directors. One questionnaire is typically used for nursing units (focused on licensed beds), another for clinical services where patients are treated within the department (focused on workload data and equipment), and another for all other support services that do not provide direct patient care (focused on staffing and processes). Baseline data are collected regarding the current scope of services, staffing and scheduling patterns, major equipment units, and workload. The perceptions of the department manager or medical director regarding current space deficiencies; workload trends; equipment suitability; and other anticipated changes in services, patient mix, processes, and technology are also solicited. Focused interviews may then be conducted to assess the ability of the department or service line to accommodate the workload forecasts and operational and technological changes identified by the planning team, as described in Chapters 3 and 4. A survey of the department's current space by an outside consultant or third party provides an objective assessment of the adequacy of current space allocation, quality of the space, equipment and procedure room utilization, and other facility planning issues.

Using Benchmarks, Rules of Thumb, and Best Practices

External validation is frequently desired through the use of industry benchmarks and rules of thumb, along with the identification of best practices at other organizations around the country. There are different types of benchmarks used in the healthcare industry, including those used to assess market demand (admissions per 1,000 population), financial performance (average cost per adjusted discharge), and labor productivity (full-time equivalents per occupied bed). For facility planning purposes, the most common types of benchmarks are those used to assess the following:

- Ability of the facilities to accommodate the current workload, such as the annual workload per treatment space

- Adequacy of overall space in a department to support the number of treatment spaces, such as the total DGSF per procedure room

- Space productivity, such as the annual procedures per DGSF

- Space efficiency, such as net-to-gross space ratios

Some examples of how benchmarks may be used to develop preliminary space estimates include the following (Hayward 2005):

- A surgery suite with 65 percent outpatient cases has 12 operating rooms (ORs) but accommodates only 9,600 annual cases (800 annual cases per OR); using a benchmark of 1,000 to 1,250 annual cases per OR, it would not need any additional ORs to accommodate the five-year growth projection of 12,500 annual cases.

- A dedicated outpatient surgery suite with six ORs currently has 15,000 DGSF (2,500 DGSF per OR), which is inadequate; using a benchmark of 2,800 DGSF per OR, it is determined that it should be allocated 16,8000 DGSF (an additional 1,800 DGSF).

Information regarding industrywide best practices, where the cost effectiveness and improved quality outcomes have been substantiated relative to different operational models, has been widely published.

Incremental Need Approach

At this stage of the space planning process, common practice is to use an *incremental need approach* versus the *zero-based budget approach* employed during the detailed functional and space programming process. With this approach, space is added or subtracted from the current space allocation to reflect specific space deficiencies and surpluses within an individual department. For example, if a respiratory therapy department is currently assigned 4,300 DGSF and has two vacant offices, then approximately 300 DGSF is subtracted from the current space allocation to arrive at the current space need of 4,000 DGSF. If at the same time this department has no temporary storage space for equipment that has been cleaned and is being held for disposition, then an estimated 100 DGSF would be added back into the current space allocation, resulting in a revised current space need of 4,100 DGSF.

These rather simple calculations are sufficient for use in preliminary space planning where the goal is to understand the magnitude of the space deficiencies by major functional category of space. The subsequent development of a detailed, room-by-room space program may result in a slightly smaller or larger space estimate for an individual department.

Scenario Analysis and Modeling

The effect of alternate workload and service configuration scenarios on space need is frequently modeled by developing appropriate assumptions and creating a computerized model or simple electronic spreadsheet. For example, Table 5.1 compares the space need for a 30-bed acute care nursing unit depending on the mix of private and semiprivate patient rooms. Compared to a nursing unit with only private patient rooms, 6 percent less space is required when 70 percent of the beds are located in private rooms, and 11 percent less space is required if 50 percent of the total beds are located in private rooms. This may not seem like a lot of space when a single nursing unit is being evaluated, particularly if the indirect operational costs are considered, such as increased patient transfers with a high number of semiprivate patient rooms. If a 200-bed replacement hospital is being planned, the difference between planning only private rooms and 70 percent of the beds in private rooms would equate to an incremental cost of $2 million to $3 million dollars.

EVALUATING FACILITY CAPACITY

Now that demand for inpatient services appears to be rising while outpatient demand continues to grow, many healthcare organizations are experiencing moderate to severe capacity constraints (AHA and

TABLE 5.1 MODELING THE SPACE NEED FOR A 30-BED NURSING UNIT

	Percent Beds in Private Rooms		
	100%	70%	50%
Number of beds in:			
Private rooms	30	22	16
Semiprivate rooms	0	4	7
Total rooms	30	26	23
Net square feet (NSF):			
Patient rooms	6,000	5,600	5,300
Toilet/shower rooms	2,580	3,120	1,380
Other support space	2,785	2,005	3,410
Total NSF	11,365	10,725	10,090
Circulation space	6,815	6,435	6,050
Department gross square feet (DGSF)	18,180	17,160	16,140
DGSF per bed	606	572	538

Lewin Group 2004). An analysis of facility capacity for clinical services involves identifying the current workload volumes and major treatment spaces and then applying industry benchmarks and rules of thumb. Evaluating the capacity of inpatient nursing units, however, is much more complicated if the organization was originally designed with a large number of multiple-bed patient rooms or has taken beds out of service at various points in time.

Even with adequate facility capacity, many healthcare organizations are limited in their weekly hours of operation because of the availability of physician, technical, and support staff—for example, scheduling difficulties, recruiting in a tight job market, and regulatory or union issues with cross-training staff. This is also true with inpatient nursing units where beds may be closed because of the inability to recruit nurses to staff them.

Bed Capacity

Any capacity assessment should begin with an inventory and analysis of the inpatient nursing units, as described in Chapter 2 and shown in Table 5.2. Inpatient nursing units are modular in design and consist of a number of patient rooms that typically share centralized support and administrative space. They vary in the number and type of patient rooms (private versus multibed), the configuration of the contiguous toilet/shower facilities, and the total DGSF used to support the specific number of beds.

As mentioned in Chapter 2, the design capacity should be identified based on physical inspection of the unit and current architectural drawings. Historically, as the census declined, many organizations began taking beds out of service and typically redeployed selected patient rooms on each unit to accommodate increasing equipment storage needs, new ancillary and clinical staff, or point-of-care services. In some cases, headwalls were removed and toilet/shower rooms reconfigured; in other cases, these features were preserved so that the rooms could be redeployed with minimal cost as demand changed. The design capacity refers to the total number of beds that could be redeployed for patient care with minimal renovation—for example, patient rooms temporarily used as offices or storage rooms with the headwalls and utilities still intact.

A review of the information displayed in Table 5.2 reveals the following:

- The nursing units located in the newer north wing have a sufficient number of private rooms (71 percent) and an ample amount of space per bed (507 DGSF). Although four of the beds on each unit are located in semiprivate rooms, with 22 patient rooms and 28 beds on each unit, the semiprivate rooms would not need to be occupied by more than one patient until the census exceeds about 80 percent.

- The older units in the south wing have minimal private rooms and an inadequate amount of space to support the staffed beds (283 to 354 DGSF per bed).

- The rehabilitation unit (4-South Wing) is particularly problematic, with only 283 DGSF per bed and no private rooms. Rehabilitation units with an extended length of stay generally require more

DGSF per bed than an acute care nursing unit to provide central dining, therapy, and family and visitor space; with all beds being in semiprivate rooms, it is unlikely that high occupancy rates could be achieved.

- Even though there is a design capacity for an additional 15 beds in the south wing, it is unlikely that former patient rooms could be redeployed given that the support space is already insufficient for the beds currently staffed.

- Although there is a severe lack of private patient rooms in the south wing, simply converting the semiprivate rooms to private rooms would not be an option because it would reduce the unit sizes such that efficient staffing patterns would not be possible—for example, a 14-bed unit.

- Compared to the medical/surgical intensive care unit (MSICU), the cardiothoracic intensive care unit (CICU) is severely undersized (364 versus 650 DGSF per bed); one of the original ten patient rooms in the CICU has already been redeployed for equipment storage.

- The mother/baby unit was originally designed with all semiprivate rooms, but 12 of the original semiprivate rooms are being used as privates because of a declining census; support space is adequate for the 20 beds currently staffed.

- The pediatric unit staffs all the original semiprivate rooms as single-bed rooms, but because of the continued low census and the shift to same-day and outpatient settings, the nine rooms are often used as an overflow for adult same-day and observation patients.

Although not shown in Table 5.2, comparison of the NSF of the patient rooms (inside wall-to-wall dimension, excluding the toilet/shower facilities and access alcove) is also useful if a variety of nursing units had been constructed or upgraded at different points in time. A review of the NSF of a typical private and semiprivate patient room on each nursing unit indicates whether an inadequate DGSF per bed ratio is a result of minimally sized patient rooms or a lack of support space, or both. Any code-compliance issues with either the size

TABLE 5.2 EXAMPLE: NURSING UNIT CAPACITY ANALYSIS

Service	Capacity Total Beds	Staffed Beds Beds	Staffed Beds Rooms	Staffed Beds in Private Rooms	Staffed Beds in Double Rooms	% Private Beds	Space DGSF	Space DGSF per Bed
General Medical/Surgical								
1-South wing (Cardiovascular)	28	24	13	2	22	8%	7,650	319
2-South wing (Medical/surgical)	28	24	14	4	20	17%	8,500	354
3-South wing (Ortho/Neuro/Urology)	30	25	15	5	20	20%	8,760	350
4-South wing (Rehab)	32	30	15	0	30	0%	8,490	283
2-North wing (Medical/surgical)	28	28	22	20	4	71%	14,200	507
3-North wing (Medical/surgical)	28	28	22	20	4	71%	14,200	507
4-North wing (Medical/surgical)	28	28	22	20	4	71%	14,200	507
Subtotal (General medical/surgical)	202	187	123	71	104	38%	76,000	406
Critical Care								
1-MSICU (Medical/surgical intensive care unit)	12	12	12	12	0	100%	7,800	650
1-CICU (Cardiothoracic intensive care unit)	10	9	9	9	0	100%	3,280	364
Subtotal (Critical care)	22	21	21	21	0	100%	11,080	528
Subtotal (Medical/surgical)	224	208	144	92	104	44%	87,080	419
Maternal/Child								
3-East (Mother/baby unit)	32	20	16	12	8	60%	9,960	498
3-West (Pediatrics/overflow adult)	18	9	9	9	9	100%	6,500	722
Subtotal (Maternal/child)	50	29	25	21	17	72%	16,460	568
Total	274	237	169	113	121	48%	103,540	437

of the patient rooms or the size and access to the contiguous patient toilet/shower facilities should also be identified.

Capacity of Major Clinical Services

It is always surprising how healthcare organizations vary in the number of expensive procedure rooms and equipment units that they use to accommodate similar numbers of annual procedures. This is why it is important to look at the current capacity of specific clinical services prior to deciding to expand the number of procedure rooms and related support space, particularly those services that use expensive equipment and require uniquely designed procedure rooms. Key questions to ask prior to committing significant dollars to expand or upgrade an existing department include the following:

- Is the current equipment state of the art? Would newer, upgraded equipment improve throughput and thus eliminate the need for additional procedure rooms? Can the current procedure rooms accommodate new, upgraded equipment, considering size and dimensions, ceiling height, floor loading capacity, and power and telecommunications requirements?

- Could the daily and weekly hours of operation be extended to allow more procedures to be performed per week with the existing or upgraded equipment, such as staffing the department during evening or weekend hours?

- Even if the current number of procedure rooms is sufficient, is support space adequate to allow the department to function efficiently and to meet customer service needs, including staff work areas; supply storage; and patient waiting, reception, preparation, and recovery space?

- Would relocating the department to an alternate location facilitate the sharing of staff, enhance customer convenience, or allow procedure rooms or support space to be shared with another department or service?

- Would a newly configured or relocated department reduce staffing costs, increase workloads and corresponding revenue, or provide other quantitative benefits that would balance the initial capital cost of equipment acquisition and facility renovation or construction?

Table 5.3 summarizes general capacity benchmarks for key diagnostic and treatment services assuming target procedure room turnaround times and moderate technology implementation. The optimal annual number of procedures that can be accommodated by a single piece of equipment or procedure room is then identified. The annual capacity is determined by first identifying the number of procedures or visits that can optimally be scheduled in an hour, as well as the number of hours per day that the department will be staffed, and then assuming 50 weeks per year of operation (allowing for about ten holidays). Some examples of factors that influence procedure room turnaround time include the following:

- *Technology.* With a traditional, single-slice CT scanner, patients were scheduled every 30 minutes such that each procedure room could accommodate 16 patient studies or procedures per day based on an eight-hour day. The newer, 16-slice scanners can acquire 32 images per second, resulting in an average procedure time of less than ten minutes. This allows four patients to be scheduled per hour, or twice the number as with the older unit.

- *Patient mix and scheduling patterns.* Physician practice space and clinics will have varying utilization of their exam rooms depending on the type of patients being seen (for example, dermatology, general surgery, oncology, and pediatrics), teaching obligations, and scheduling patterns such as evening and weekend sessions.

- *Responsiveness of support services.* The time required to prepare a surgical OR for the next case (OR turnover time) has a significant impact on the daily number of cases that can be accommodated in a single operating room.

- *Responsiveness of other hospital departments.* The turnaround of ED exam and treatment cubicles is greatly influenced by the responsiveness of the central laboratory and imaging departments if point-of-care services are not available; the responsiveness of consulting physicians also affects patient throughput in the ED.

Physician Practice Space and Outpatient Clinics

Physician practice space was traditionally planned assuming two exam rooms and an office/consultation room for each physician. The space

TABLE 5.3 CAPACITY BENCHMARKS FOR MAJOR DIAGNOSTIC TREATMENT SERVICES

Service/ Workload Unit	Category	Average Annual Workload per Treatment Space	Average DGSF per Treatment Space
Emergency visits	ED treatment	1,300 to 1,700	550 to 650
	Fast track treatment	1,700 to 2,400	400 to 450
Surgery cases	Inpatients primarily	800 to 900	2,400 to 2,500
	Inpatient/outpatient mix	1,000 to 1,250	2,500 to 2,800
	Outpatient suite	1,250 to 1,500	2,800 to 3,000
Obstetrical births	LDRP exclusively	100 to 200	800 to 1,000
	LDR primarily	300 to 400	
Cardiology procedures	Diagnostic catheterization	1,200 to 1,800	2,000 to 2,400
	Electrophysiology	600 to 900	2,000 to 2,400
	Noninvasive	2,000 to 2,400	500 to 900
Imaging procedures	General rad/fluoro	6,000 to 7,000	1,300 to 1,500
	Computed tomography	8,000 to 9,000	1,800 to 2,000
	Mammography	5,500 to 6,000	1,000 to 1,200
	Magnetic resonance	4,000 to 6,000	2,200 to 3,000
	Nuclear medicine/PET	2,200 to 2,500	1,800 to 2,000
	Angiography	1,200 to 1,800	2,000 to 2,400
	Ultrasound	4,000 to 4,500	900 to 1,200
Special procedures	Endoscopy	1,250 to 1,500	800 to 1,200
Radiation oncology visits	Linear accelerator	8,000 to 10,000	6,000 to 7,000
	Chemotherapy/infusions	500 to 1,000	250 to 350
Physician office visits	Private physician office	2,400 to 4,500	400 to 450
	Faculty/resident clinic	1,000 to 2,000	450 to 600

Source: Hayward, C. 2005. SpaceMed—A Space Planning Guide for Healthcare Facilities. Ann Arbor, MI: Hayward & Associates, LLC. [Online information; retrieved 7/21/05.] www.space-med.com.

was dedicated for use by a specific physician, regardless of the hours per week that he or she was present. Because of the competing responsibilities of most physicians, including seeing inpatients, performing surgery and other procedures, seeing outpatients in other locations, and attending conferences, only a portion of the total physicians generally used their allocated exam rooms at a given time. Exam rooms were typically underutilized on Monday mornings and Fridays while experiencing peak demand during mid-week. The variance between peak-volume and low-volume days is even more pronounced in academic medical centers where medical faculty also have teaching and research responsibilities that further reduce (and affect the scheduling of) their time in outpatient clinics.

The space needed for physician practices and outpatient clinics is usually planned based on the anticipated schedule and staffing patterns. Two exam rooms per provider are typically planned, although high-volume, quick-turnaround specialties, such as dermatology and orthopedics, may effectively use three exam rooms per provider. However, the weekly number of visits per exam room should also be calculated to identify whether exam rooms are being fully utilized. For example, 400 visits per week (Monday through Friday, eight hours per day) with 24 exam rooms result in an average of 3.3 visits per exam room per day. If patients are typically scheduled two per hour in a particular clinic, a utilization factor of only 21 percent results. In this case, alteration of the planned scheduling pattern should be considered so that fewer half-day clinic sessions per week are scheduled, resulting in the potential reassignment of the exam rooms to another provider team during other times of the week.

Providers typically schedule a range of one to four patients per hour. This depends on the specialty and the proportion of new patient visits versus return or follow-up visits, which affects the length of time that the patient spends in the exam room. I generally use an exam room utilization factor of 90 percent for private practitioners who do not have a high number of no-show patients. Teaching clinics, where care is provided primarily by residents supervised by academic physicians (who together spend longer times with patients) and where there is a large number of no-shows, typically see the fewest number of patients per exam room per day. In this case, an exam room utilization factor of 70 percent would be used for planning purposes.

Well-planned physician practice space and outpatient clinics provide sufficient intrinsic flexibility to accommodate sizable deviations from workload forecasts. This is accomplished by creating spaces that can be used interchangeably for various types of visits; by understanding the relationships among workload, service times, and staffing to respond to unexpected surges in workload; and by accommodating a wide range of patient visits in a single flexible exam or treatment space. For example, if ten patients are typically seen per exam room per day, extending the daily schedule to 7 p.m. allows the same space to accommodate a 25 percent increase in annual workload. Moreover, using the exam rooms to see patients for eight hours on Saturday increases the weekly capacity by another 20 percent (48 hours per week versus 40 hours).

UNDERSTANDING YOUR OUTPATIENT POPULATION

The explosion of outpatient growth in the 1980s and 1990s, coupled with an intense focus on patient convenience, led to a proliferation of dedicated and freestanding outpatient facilities on and off campus. Unfortunately, it has been my observation that some new outpatient facilities resulted in increased operational costs with little incremental revenue to support the redundant staff, equipment, and space. A healthcare organization should understand its current outpatient population before embarking on facility master planning. This requires at least an initial analysis of how many and what types of outpatients come to the hospital campus on a typical day, in addition to their specific destinations; an example of this type of analysis is shown in Figure 5.1. Typical daily outpatient visits can be estimated by dividing the annual workload by the annual days of operation of the specific service and then applying a factor to account for scheduling variations throughout the week and by shift, as applicable. For example, you can generally assume that 10 percent to 20 percent more patients will visit the campus on the peak weekday than on the average. In the case of the ED, you can assume that 50 percent of the estimated daily emergency visits will occur on the busiest shift.

BENCHMARKING YOUR CURRENT FUNCTIONAL LAYOUT AGAINST TEN FACILITY CONFIGURATION PRINCIPLES

You can perform a mini-assessment of the current functional layout of your facilities and identify potential issues by comparing your current

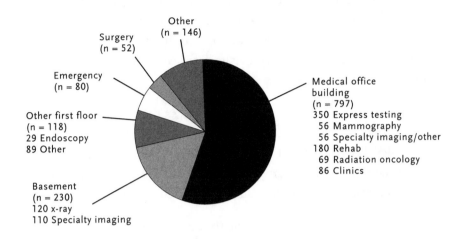

Other
(n = 146)

Surgery
(n = 52)

Emergency
(n = 80)

Other first floor
(n = 118)
29 Endoscopy
89 Other

Medical office
building
(n = 797)
350 Express testing
 56 Mammography
 56 Specialty imaging/other
180 Rehab
 69 Radiation oncology
 86 Clinics

Basement
(n = 230)
120 x-ray
110 Specialty imaging

site and facilities to the following ten optimal configuration principles:

1. *Separate key types of campus traffic.* Site access points should be clearly marked with directional signage to relevant parking lots and easily identifiable building entrance points for emergency traffic, service traffic, and public and visitor traffic heading for patient intake and admission, medical office buildings, or various outpatient services. External signage should be reviewed with the fresh eyes of someone who is unfamiliar with the specific campus to identify issues relative to misleading, incomprehensible, or inconsistent destination names and directional signs that are unreadable or absent.

2. *Clearly define the front door.* Just as most shopping centers are designed with a single prominent entrance to assist first-time customers who are unfamiliar with the overall layout and require orientation, large healthcare centers should have a clearly defined front door, even though patients may be encouraged to go directly to their service destination on subsequent visits.

3. *Coordinate and collocate customer intake and access services.* A single, one-stop shopping location (such as a customer service center, for patient and visitor reception; information dissemination; intake and access functions, including admitting, registration, and insurance verification; family support services; and amenities) should be provided, generally adjacent to the front door and from which other patient and visitor services can be coordinated (hub-and-spoke concept).

4. *Optimize the use of prime real estate.* Services that involve customer interaction and face-to-face contact should be concentrated on the grade-level floor adjacent to the front door. The use of this prime real estate for administrative offices and other support services that could be located remote should be discouraged.

5. *Minimize the total number of outpatient destinations.* Related clinical services should be grouped around a centralized reception and intake area or other destination marked with clear and consistent directional signage; patients are then escorted to the point of care when the staff and procedure room are available. Diagramming the current number of possible outpatient destinations and the routes required to reach them also identifies inconvenient service locations and wayfinding issues.

6. *Position diagnostic and treatment services for changing technology and future operational flexibility* by collocating services with similar facility needs such as the following:

   - Routine, quick-turnaround procedures—for example, phlebotomy and simple x-rays

   - Specialty imaging, interventional services, and surgery

   - Same-day medical procedures

7. *Minimize inpatient transfers* by providing private patient rooms (to the extent possible), organizing inpatient nursing units by specialty rather that acuity (depending on volumes), and implementing the acuity-adaptable patient room concept (where possible).

8. *Unbundle high-volume, recurring outpatient services to an off-site location.* If contiguous parking and convenient access cannot be

achieved on the main campus, high-volume, recurring, outpatient services should be relocated off site; examples include outpatient physical therapy, outpatient behavioral health, and outpatient dialysis.

9. *Unbundle building support services.* Space for building support services should be located in inexpensive construction (on or off site) while facilitating efficient material distribution to key users such as inpatient nursing units.

10. *Provide flexible, generic administrative office space.* Larger office suites should be planned (on or off site) in lieu of smaller pockets of offices throughout the hospital campus; flexible, generic office space should be planned to accommodate various department staff who do not require face-to-face contact with customers; offices and workstations can be reassigned periodically as programs and staffing levels change.

SUMMARIZING SPACE REQUIREMENTS

Using each department's footprint, a comparison should be made between the current space allocation, the current space need (based on current services, workload, and resources), and the future space need (based on program growth, new services, and anticipated operational and technological changes). Space should be organized and subtotaled by the major functional categories discussed in Chapter 2. The planning horizon should correspond to the workload forecasts (typically five years), and multiple scenarios may be modeled to reflect various assumptions regarding bed need and ancillary workloads. In addition, space efficiencies that could be achieved by consolidating departments either on site or off site should be identified. The future space projections should be based on a foundation of supporting data and an objective assessment of actual need rather than solely on department or service-line manager perceptions.

SUMMARIZING KEY FACILITY ISSUES AND ESTABLISHING PRIORITIES

Because it may not be practical to solve all facility problems within a given planning horizon, the importance of individual problems must be evaluated in relation to one another. To make facility decisions, an organization must be able to understand both the magnitude and relative urgency of facility problems as they pertain to strategic planning, operations improvement, and technology investment initiatives. Facility planning issues and current space deficiencies can be summarized in a matrix format so that departments and service lines can be readily prioritized relative to the urgency with which the deficiencies need to be resolved. Figure 5.2 presents an example of a matrix that summarizes key facility issues and presents them in a concise manner to facilitate setting priorities during the facility planning process. The matrix is utilized to evaluate all departments and service lines against a common set of criteria. These criteria range from operational concerns to questions of department location, internal layout, and finally to specific physical plant considerations. Evaluation criteria can be separated into overall facility planning issues and specific space deficiencies. Facility planning issues for most hospital departments include the following:

- *Workload capacity issues.* The current facilities cannot accommodate recent workload growth, or a surplus capacity exists.

- *Operational/process issues.* Inappropriate policies prevent the efficient scheduling of patients and staff.

- *Poor functional layout.* The layout of the internal department impedes smooth and efficient workflow.

- *Inappropriate location.* The space and functional layout may be adequate, but the location is remote from related patient and support services.

- *Equipment/technology issues.* Equipment is outdated or unreliable, or archaic IT systems are still employed.

- *Poor image/interior design.* The furnishings are worn out, and the interior décor is outdated.

- *Physical plant/environmental issues.* There are temperature control problems, electrical shortages, plumbing leaks, vibrations, etc.

- *Code/regulatory issues.* Code noncompliances have been cited by regulatory agencies, and a plan for rectification must be developed.

Each of the potential issues listed above has very different cost and timing implications for the organization.

Space issues can be evaluated relative to deficiencies with the following:

- *Patient rooms too small* to provide quality patient care, incorporate new equipment and technology, accommodate family members and visitors

- *Lack of diagnostic and treatment space* to support the current workload, provide an appropriate work environment for physicians and technicians, and accommodate new equipment and technology

- *Lack of staff/administrative space*, such as staff workstations, offices, lounges, toilet/shower facilities, and conference rooms

- *Lack of other support space*, such as clean and soiled utility rooms and equipment storage space

- *Inadequate customer intake space and amenities*, including reception; registration; waiting areas; and other amenities such as phones, toilet/shower facilities, and food service

Additional issues related to inpatient nursing units (also shown in Figure 5.2) include a lack of private patient rooms, inadequate toilet/shower facilities, and the size of the patient room.

The types of facility issues and space deficiencies have different implications as well. Inappropriately sized and configured treatment areas with outdated equipment and technology may affect the quality of care and increase medical errors, while inadequate staff workstations may negatively affect staff recruiting and retention. Undersized and inappropriate patient and visitor support space, a lack of amenities, and outdated interior décor and furnishings may promote a negative first impression among the organization's customers and defeat efforts to increase volumes and expand market share.

FIGURE 5.2   EXAMPLE: SUMMARIZING KEY FACILITY ISSUES

Nursing Units

Facility Planning Issues

Nursing Unit	Poor functional layout	Inappropriate location	Inappropriate traffic mix	Lack of private rooms	Inadequate toilet facilities	Inadequate bathing facilities	Poor image/ interior design	Physical plant/ environmental issues	Code/regulatory issues
2-West (Medical/surgical)			●	●		●			
2-South (Orthopedics)								●	
3-West (Rehabilitation)							◉		

Space Deficiencies

Nursing Unit	Patient rooms too small	Lack of staff/ administrative space	Lack of other support space	Inadequate patient/ visitor amenities
2-West (Medical/surgical)				●
2-South (Orthopedics)			●	
3-West (Rehabilitation)	●	◉		

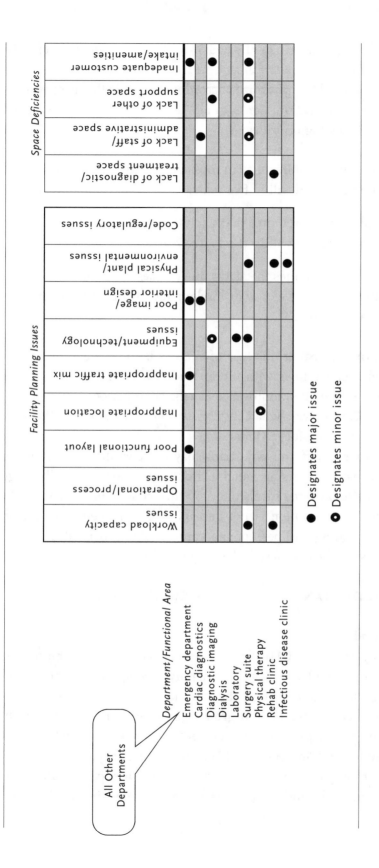

As each department is evaluated against a common set of criteria, major versus minor issues may be further delineated. Finally, each department should be prioritized according to a scale that is relevant to the specific organization. For example, departments may be assigned one of the following priorities:

- High priority requires that an immediate solution be developed and implemented within two years.

- Medium priority requires that a solution be developed and implemented within two to five years.

- Low priority assumes the status quo or does not need for a solution to be developed or implemented within a five-year planning horizon.

The primary goal of this type of analysis is to separate the departments and service lines with more critical facility issues from those that require little attention over a specific time period—for example, five years. This allows the facility planning effort to proceed efficiently and in a logical and focused manner.

Department staff and physicians may perceive that their facilities are inadequate for reasons ranging from equipment and technology deficiencies to outdated furnishings to actual code noncompliances. In many cases, the solution is not necessarily an updated or expanded facility. Separating staff perceptions from actual facility needs is critical to a successful facility master planning process.

CASE STUDY: PLANNING A MULTISPECIALTY CLINIC

Background

University Hospital (UH) planned to consolidate several outpatient clinics into a single, efficient ambulatory care space in a new, free-standing building. Although the current number of annual visits (30,000) was not expected to grow significantly in the near future, three different locations were currently in operation, which was perceived to result in operational and space inefficiencies.

One of the goals was to reduce the number of support staff, along with patient intake and reception space, by consolidating all visits into a single location. However, the faculty leadership debated the planning approach for the new facility. Some wished to maintain the status quo, while others recognized that reducing their staff and facility costs would improve profitability while potentially improving customer service with more streamlined and better coordinated processes. The physician leadership agreed to evaluate the impact on overall space need and resulting construction cost of planning a "lean" facility versus a more "generous" facility.

Planning Approach

A number of factors were identified that would ultimately affect the overall size of the new clinic facility. These are illustrated in Table 5.4 and include the following:

- *Annual visits per exam room.* Currently, the three clinics average only 1,000 annual visits per exam room. By extending clinic hours to early evening (and possibly Saturday) and by leveling out the scheduling of physician and resident clinic sessions during the week, a target of 1,650 annual visits per exam room was deemed appropriate.

- *Number of exam rooms.* A total of 30 exam rooms were currently used at the three locations; only 18 exam rooms would be needed if annual visits per exam room were increased.

- *Exam rooms per module.* Two modules of nine exam rooms each, versus the current clinic configuration of four modules with six to eight exam rooms per module, were considered for the new facility. Using two modules in lieu of the current four results in a reduction of the overall DNSF by providing shared patient intake and reception space, staff amenities, and other support space.

- *NSF per exam room.* Alternate exam room layouts were considered as the clinic standard, ranging from a more compact exam room with 95 NSF to a more spacious exam room with 120 NSF.

- *DGSF to NSF ratio.* Alternate clinic layouts with varying amounts of DGSF to accommodate the projected NSF were evaluated. The higher ratio assumed wider internal corridors and a facility layout that required an additional egress corridor.

TABLE 5.4 PLANNING CLINIC SPACE FOR 30,000 ANNUAL VISITS

	Lean	Generous
	30,000	**30,000**
Annual visits per exam room	1,650	1,000
Number of exam rooms	18	30
Exam rooms per module	8 to 12	6 to 8
Net square feet (NSF) per exam room	95	120
Total department NSF	4,900	11,400
Total NSF to DGSF ratio	1.30	1.45
Department gross square feet (DGSF)	6,400	16,500
BGSF to DGSF ratio	1.20	1.30
Building gross square feet (BGSF)	7,700	21,500
Annual visits per BGSF	3.9	1.4

Source: Hayward, C. 2005. *SpaceMed—A Space Planning Guide for Healthcare Facilities*. Ann Arbor, MI: Hayward & Associates, LLC. [Online information; retrieved 7/21/05.] www.space-med.com.

- *BGSF to DGSF ratio*. Alternate architectural designs with varying amounts of total BGSF, or overall building footprint, to accommodate the same DGSF were evaluated. The higher ratio assumed a large atrium, more generous elevator lobby, and a larger mechanical equipment room.

- *Annual visits per BGSF*. The resulting annual visits per total BGSF varied from 3.9 in the lean model to only 1.4 in the generous model.

Conclusion

Assuming an overall project cost of approximately $250 per BGSF, the generous approach would require $3.5 million more (almost three times as much) to construct the new clinic facility than would the lean approach.

CASE STUDY: EVALUATING ED EXPANSION

Background

Midwest Hospital (MH) planned to expand and potentially replace its ED in response to increased crowding and congestion. Although the current number of annual visits (40,000) was not expected to grow significantly in the near future, the patient and visitor waiting room was frequently overflowing during the evening hours. ED staff also began creating "hall beds" by labeling and assigning defined stretcher bays in the hallways to gain additional treatment space during peak periods. The relocation of an adjacent occupational medicine clinic was viewed as an option for ED expansion in lieu of total ED replacement.

Specific facility expansion goals included expanding the patient and visitor waiting space with enhanced amenities; providing adequate exam and treatment space; triaging nonurgent patients in a separate, fast-track area; and developing a holding area for patients to be admitted who are waiting for an available inpatient bed. Although facility expansion and operations improvement were deemed necessary by all members of the planning team, the CFO was concerned about spending significant capital dollars when ED revenues were relatively flat. ED staff were also not in agreement regarding the extent of required expansion; some wanted to almost double the size of the current ED, while others were concerned that significant expansion would require additional staff at a time when budgets were tight and recruiting was difficult. Others were concerned about the long ED length of stay and its impact on customer satisfaction. However, all members of the planning team agreed that a detailed analysis of the relationship between improvements in exam and treatment room turnaround time and resulting space need and construction cost was warranted prior to initiating the detailed operational and space programming process.

Planning Approach

A detailed database was assembled, and a number of operational issues were identified that would ultimately affect the overall size of the upgraded ED as follows:

- *Trend in ED utilization and patient mix.* Historically, emergency visits at MH increased 2 percent to 4 percent annually; however, ED visits have stabilized at around 40,000 annual visits during the past two years. The leveling-off in volume has been generally attributed to a communitywide initiative to redirect the uninsured to primary care clinics. However, MH's ED has been on diversion frequently because of a lack of intensive care beds at the hospital. Both the percentage of ED patients that are admitted (currently at 18 percent) and the percentage of nonurgent care patients (currently at 40 percent) have been increasing, even though total ED volume has stabilized.

- *Treatment room turnaround time.* Currently, the average treatment room turnaround time at MH is more than three hours, or 180 minutes, which is even longer when the time from initial triage to placement in the treatment room and the time from exiting the treatment room to eventual discharge are added. Critical operational issues include slow responsiveness from the imaging department for CT scans, lengthy test report turnaround time from the central laboratory, and long waiting times for physician consultations. The backup in the ED of patients to be admitted while they are waiting for an available inpatient bed is also a major issue.

- *Number of treatment bays.* A total of 29 ED treatment spaces are currently available, including two large triage and resuscitation rooms and dedicated rooms for obstetrics-gynecology and orthopedic casting. Four of the treatment bays are designated for nonurgent patients, although they are generally used on a first-come-first-serve basis with no formal fast-track procedure in place. In addition, a dedicated x-ray room is located within the ED, resulting in a total of 30 patient treatment and procedure spaces.

- *Average NSF per treatment bay.* The existing treatment room or bay currently averages only 105 NSF, with some stretcher bays sized at less than 70 NSF compared to contemporary standards of 120 NSF for general ED treatment rooms; more than double the space is required for trauma and resuscitation rooms.

- *Total DGSF per treatment room/bay ratio.* The ratio of the current amount of DGSF to the total number of treatment and procedure rooms (or bays) was evaluated to assess the adequacy of the overall footprint of the ED to support the current number of treatment rooms and bays. With 11,250 DGSF occupied by the current ED, an average of 375 DGSF per treatment space is calculated compared to contemporary design standards of 550 to 650 DGSF per treatment or procedure space. This indicates a severe shortage of support space and inadequately sized treatment cubicles.

- *Average annual visits per treatment bay.* With 40,000 annual ED visits and 30 treatment bays and rooms, MH currently accommodates 1,333 annual ED visits per treatment room/bay.

Effect of Treatment Room Turnaround Time on ED Space and Project Costs

An overview analysis of the impact of treatment room turnaround time on required ED treatment rooms, total DGSF, and total project cost was performed. The analysis revealed that even minor improvements in ED turnaround time would have a significant effect on the space and resulting renovation or construction costs, as shown in Table 5.5.

Conclusion

Because of the high cost of replacing the existing ED, particularly if 30 or more treatment cubicles and support space were provided, the ED planning team ultimately decided to focus their operations improvement efforts on improving ED treatment room turnaround time to a target of 120 minutes before embarking on a major renovation or construction project.

Because the adjacent occupational health clinic (with six exam rooms and support space) schedules patients only on Monday through Friday and is typically closed at 4:00 p.m. each day, and because ED demand for nonurgent (fast-track) space is typically from 4:00 p.m. until 11:00 p.m., an operational plan was developed to use the occupational health clinic's space to triage and treat nonurgent ED patients

TABLE 5.5 IMPACT OF TREATMENT ROOM TURNAROUND TIME ON ED SPACE
AND PROJECT COST

Average Treatment Bay Turnaround Time	Treatment Bays Required	Gross Space Required at 550 to 650 DGSF/Room	Estimated Project Cost
90 minutes	20	11,000 to 13,000 DGSF	$3.9 to $4.6 Million
120 minutes	25	13,750 to 16,250 DGSF	$4.8 to $5.7 Million
180 minutes	35	19,250 to 22,750 DGSF	$6.8 to $8.0 Million

Source: Hayward, C. 2005. *SpaceMed—A Space Planning Guide for Healthcare Facilities.* Ann Arbor, MI: Hayward & Associates, LLC. [Online information; retrieved 7/21/05.] www.space-med.com.

during the evenings and on weekends. With the diversion of these nonurgent patients out of the main ED, the smallest ED treatment rooms and bays were reconfigured, resulting in 25 appropriately sized ED treatment rooms and cubicles in addition to the six fast-track exam and treatment rooms. A modest expansion of the patient and family waiting area was undertaken using adjacent office space. This interim solution allowed MH to monitor trends in ED volume and evaluate the success of its operations improvement efforts. Hospital leadership agreed to reevaluate the need for a major ED expansion or replacement project again in another year.

SPECIFIC ISSUES ASSOCIATED WITH ELIMINATING SURPLUS CAPACITY

Much effort was spent over the past two decades to eliminate surplus capacity in response to declining inpatient admissions and length of stay; overbuilt outpatient facilities; shrinking hospital-based diagnostic and treatment departments; and oversized building support space—such as the laundry, warehouse, and kitchen—that was originally designed for a much larger hospital chassis at a time when hospitals provided all services on site. Although the number of hospital mergers has been falling steadily since 1996, consolidation is continuing, just not at the pace observed in the mid-1990s (Guerin-Calvert et al. 2003). Regardless, newly merged multihospital healthcare systems must still deal with redundant services and surplus capacity. Realigning services and reallocating resources among multiple campuses require a unique strategic, operations improvement, and facility planning process. Alternate ways of allocating resources should be thoroughly evaluated and the impact on operational costs fully understood prior to spending money on bricks and mortar. Multihospital healthcare systems also need to understand the market and patient population served at each of the individual hospital campuses. A different facility planning approach is required when two or more campuses, or sites, share the same market versus when they have distinctly separate markets. Planning at the service-line level is also required because some service lines may share the same market and others may not.

Although there are many opportunities to eliminate surplus capacity, the following key areas represent the most significant opportunities.

Eliminating Empty Beds

Although consolidating occupied beds into larger nursing units and closing or converting complete floors of beds to an alternate use can have some impact on operational costs, the real cost savings occur when entire hospitals are closed. The dramatic reduction in inpatient length of stay over the last several decades has not been because all the patients who traditionally occupied acute care beds were being treated in freestanding outpatient facilities or were simply being discharged from the hospital and sent home sooner. Same-day or short stays have increased, and this growing group of acute ambulatory (short-stay) patients are often sicker and less ambulatory than traditional outpatients, even though their hospital stays may not exceed 24 hours. Conversion of some surplus acute care bed capacity for same-day stay patients or post-acute services may be an option depending on the overall condition of the infrastructure and code compliance of the facility.

Integrating and Restructuring Clinical Services

Historically, hospitals have had a reputation for being inefficient and compartmentalized, with high overhead and inflexible full-time employees. Departmental turf wars for real estate, resources, and supplies are still common. These problems only get worse when two hospitals try to merge their operations. However, the rationale for a merger between two or more hospitals is often stated as something like this: "The new health-care environment demands a leaner, downsized, more nimble, bottom-line oriented business enterprise." Opportunities to reduce surplus capacity through clinical service integration include the following:

- Consolidating expensive diagnostic and treatment services

- Identifying the lowest cost and most appropriate setting to deliver outpatient and chronic or recurring care

- Evaluating extended hours of operation in lieu of equipment acquisition and more space to further improve utilization of resources

- Investigating the center of excellence or "institute" concept as an alternative to traditional organizational models

- Restructuring routine, high-volume, quick-turnaround testing to improve patient access and to cross-utilize staffing and space

Consolidating Physician Practices

As more physician practices become part of larger specialty groups, opportunities arise to reduce operating costs by sharing resources. Some opportunities include sharing reception and registration, waiting space, and other patient and staff amenities; sharing of support staff, thus reducing the need for offices and workstations; and sharing specialized staff, expensive treatment and special procedure rooms, and diagnostic facilities. The number of exam rooms can also be reduced by improved utilization through time sharing and planning more generic, flexible space.

Reducing Building Support Space

Most of today's hospitals were designed with a chassis to support a much larger number of inpatient beds than are currently being occupied. Space for support services is commonly located in the basement, or below-grade. When two organizations merge, the surplus space further increases. Many multihospital systems have implemented the *mosaic approach* by designating specific campuses for consolidation of specific services, thus reducing the investment in duplicate and redundant resources. For example, a single kitchen may be located at one site (with the cook-chill system used to deliver food to the remaining sites) and a single warehouse located at another site from which supplies are distributed.

Remembering that Nature Abhors a Vacuum

When there is ample surplus space, hospital departments tend to metastasize into the space available, whether or not all the space is needed. This leads to a lack of appreciation for space as an important asset by the users, and it may result in an exaggerated space allocation when the department is relocated to leased space or an alternate facility and the incremental need approach is used to estimate the size of the new space.

Separating Major Consolidation Issues from Nonissues

Paralysis often sets in when recently merged institutions begin consolidation planning. Assuming that market dynamics and demographics have been carefully considered, the key is to quickly separate actual facility consolidation issues from nonissues. Questions that should be initially addressed when considering the consolidation of one or more acute care hospitals at a single site include the following:

- Are there contemporary inpatient nursing units in a modern physical plant with code-compliant, appropriately sized patient rooms and adjoining toilet/shower facilities? What percent of the beds are in private patient rooms? How many total patient "rooms" are available?

- Are surgical operating rooms, including open-heart, updated and adequately sized? What is the capacity considering extended hours of operation?

- Are there contemporary obstetrical labor/delivery facilities? What is the capacity assuming that a single-room maternity model may not be achievable?

- What is the size and number of specialty imaging procedure rooms for procedures such as MRI, CT, angiography, cardiac catheterization, and radiation therapy? Is the technology state of the art?

- What is the customer's first impression of each facility? Is there convenient patient access, adequate parking, and a welcoming entrance lobby? Is the facility surrounded by green space, or is it a land-locked site with adversarial neighbors?

- Is there room on the site for building or parking expansion?

- What is the amount, proximity, and ownership of specialty physician offices on each site, particularly if one site will potentially be abandoned?

Less important issues that are often given more attention than warranted include diagnostic and treatment services that do not involve large fixed equipment or require specific design requirements—for example, ultrasound and physical therapy—and any department whose space is primarily offices and workstations versus clinical and patient care space.

In the mid-1990s, nearly two out of every five hospitals in the United States were involved in mergers, acquisitions, or joint ventures (Cochrane 1997). However, my experience with multihospital systems indicates that the urgency to eliminate surplus capacity and to achieve the corresponding operational cost savings often coincides with when the health system runs out of cash and debt capacity.

Russ Coile (1997) observed that "Deeply entrenched economic interests and local politics are serious considerations which any health-care executive must overcome when recommending consolidation or closure." He cited a number of political and emotional factors, including regulatory issues and the involvement of state attorneys general; community opposition and public relations problems; displaced workers, unions, and the economic impact on the community; and the effect on local philanthropy when a hospital is closed. Abandoning facilities with new additions or recently renovated space creates both emotional and political issues. Physician ownership of office space and diagnostic facilities on or near a hospital site to be abandoned further complicates the equation. The opportunities for cost savings, however, are tremendous. Funds used to support surplus capacity could be deployed for a long list of alternate purposes, including the eventual replacement of the core physical plant and technology of the surviving institutions. Unfortunately, funds spent on postponing the inevitable will not be available for investing in the future, and decisions to fund operating losses are rarely evaluated relative to the lost opportunity.

REFERENCES

American Hospital Association (AHA) and Lewin Group. 2004. *TrendWatch Chartbook 2004: Trends Affecting Hospitals and Health Systems.* Chicago: American Hospital Association.

Cochrane, J. D. 1997. "Healthcare Megatrends." *Integrated Healthcare Review* (5) 1: 1–16.

Coile, R. C., Jr., and C. Hayward. 1997. "Excess Hospital Capacity." *Russ Coile's Health Trends* (10) 1: 1–4.

Guerin-Calvert, M. E., A. Argue, P. Godek, B. Harris, and S. Mirrow. 2003. *Economic Analysis of Healthcare Cost Studies Commissioned by the American Hospital Association and Blue Cross Blue Shield Association.* Report. Chicago: American Hospital Association.

Hayward, C. 2005. *SpaceMed—A Space Planning Guide for Healthcare Facilities.* Ann Arbor, MI: Hayward & Associates, LLC. [Online information; retrieved 7/21/05.] http://www.space-med.com.

CHAPTER SIX

Reaching Consensus on a Long-Range Facility Investment Strategy

I N THE TRADITIONAL facility master planning process, facility deficiencies and future space projections are often translated directly into facility "options" that are represented by architectural drawings. A preferred design solution is subsequently selected. Renovation or construction cost estimates and a phased construction schedule are developed, with individual projects identified for funding approval and staged implementation. As part of the implementation of the facility master plan, the design architect is then commissioned to provide more detailed architectural drawings and to prepare construction documents.

The problem with this approach is that alternative operational concepts are often evaluated (if evaluated at all!) based on an architectural rendering rather than on sound business principles and consistency with specific strategic planning and operations improvement objectives. For example, alternative surgery suite configurations, such as a combined inpatient/outpatient suite versus a separate outpatient surgery suite, may be drawn by the architect when such a decision should be made prior to the design process and should be based on an evaluation of case mix and workload volumes, operational costs, surgeon preferences and revenue generation, and customer access. This kind of facility master planning process, where the planning team jumps prematurely into design with the sole output being an architectural block drawing of planned future department locations and building projects, is no longer relevant given the dynamic health-care industry. If market conditions change and workload projections do not come to fruition or if department leadership changes such that one or more projects prove infeasible, the entire plan is deemed outdated and shelved.

WHY DEVELOP A LONG-RANGE FACILITY INVESTMENT STRATEGY?

The gap between the identification of facility deficiencies and future space needs, and the subsequent architectural solutions, should be bridged with a thorough evaluation of priorities and capital investment trade-offs. Consensus on the resulting long-range facility development strategy, or "capital investment strategy," allows the planning team to begin a phased implementation of the facility master plan with confidence. They can readily alter their course as needed to reflect unanticipated changes in the market, reimbursement, regulations, and technology.

The long-range facility investment strategy essentially provides a road map to guide renovation and construction (and capital investment) over a defined planning horizon. It helps senior leadership to understand key facility issues and priorities facing the organization and to reach consensus on capital investment goals and objectives. It also aligns facility investments with the organization's strategic (market) plan, operations improvement initiatives, planned IT invest-ments (IT strategic plan), and financial resources. Documentation of an agreed-on facility investment strategy assists in the education of physicians, employees, and other stakeholders relative to long-range planning goals and priorities. Unlike the traditional facility master plan, adherence to defined strategies allows for a dynamic process that does not become obsolete if one or more individual projects are derailed.

COMMON STRATEGIES DEVELOPED BY HEALTHCARE ORGANIZATIONS TODAY

From my experience, the most common facility investment strategies developed by healthcare organizations generally involve the following:

- Bed allocation and nursing unit reconfiguration

- Clinical services reconfiguration and upgrading

- Outpatient services configuration and provision of physician office space

- Building infrastructure upgrading and equipment acquisition/replacement

- Patient experience improvement

Bed Allocation and Nursing Unit Reconfiguration

Today, much of the costly inpatient care in the United States is still delivered in facilities that were designed when cost-based reimbursement was the norm, nurses were easy to recruit, and the nurse-call system was considered "high-tech." Inpatient care is often fragmented into small, specialized units organized by acuity level, with much of the care delivered by specialists from large, centralized ancillary departments. Simple patient care activities, such as a chest x-ray or a blood test, may require numerous steps and personnel, resulting in prolonged turnaround times, delayed decision making, extended lengths of stay, and ultimately increased costs. Along with a high number of semiprivate patient rooms, this results in frequent patient transfers that involve multiple departments and staff throughout the organization. After being encouraged over the past two decades to reduce surplus inpatient bed capacity in response to declining admissions, use rates, and lengths of stay, some hospitals are struggling to accommodate growing inpatient volumes, particularly high-acuity patients.

Because of the large amount of space devoted to inpatient care in the typical hospital, with inpatient care representing a disproportionately large percentage of an organization's total costs, healthcare organizations with aging facilities need to develop a strategy for reconfiguring inefficient nursing units, updating outdated facilities, and in some cases expanding or replacing beds. A long-range facility reconfiguration plan should address inpatient nursing unit configuration by service line, acuity, and type of patient accommodation—private, semiprivate, short-stay, or observation—and should correspond to anticipated high-bed and low-bed scenarios. For healthcare organizations with inadequate accommodations for high-acuity patients, a limited number of private rooms, and aging facilities, a phased plan for ongoing bed replacement is necessary. Potential bed expansion must also be addressed in growing and aging markets.

As discussed in Chapter 3, identifying the range of beds that may be needed and then developing a flexible facility investment strategy that can be adjusted as certain benchmarks are achieved are important for facility planning purposes. Specific strategies may involve the following:

- Constructing additional new beds to meet the high-bed scenario, or replacing some of the existing, outdated beds with new beds if the high-bed scenario turns out to be overly aggressive

- Constructing larger acuity-adaptable patient rooms, with some of the rooms having the capability to accommodate two patients if the bed-need projection is underestimated or to accommodate seasonal fluctuations in census

- Redeploying existing patient rooms as either privates or semiprivates to offset inaccuracies in projecting future demand

- Developing a day recovery or observation unit that is both less expensive and quicker to construct than a traditional inpatient nursing unit to supplement inpatient bed need

Clinical Services Reconfiguration and Upgrading

Healthcare organizations are reconfiguring and often realigning clinical services among multiple locations at increasing rates. Such plans should be based on a formal, well-conceived strategy to enhance customer access, to reduce operational costs, and to minimize ongoing capital investments by planning flexible, multiuse space. Although future expansion may be planned for EDs or interventional imaging services, many hospital-based departments are being downsized because of the shift of treatments and procedures to the point of care. With increasingly miniaturized and mobile equipment, such as table-top lab test analyzers and portable digital imaging units, and the gravitation of services to the physicians' office as equipment becomes less costly to acquire, such as ultrasound and EKG, large, centralized departments need to be reconfigured. With the high cost of the most advanced, floor-mounted imaging equipment, such as high-speed CT and PET scanners, departments are often expected to schedule patients on extended shifts and weekends, thus increasing their workload capacity significantly without increasing their space.

Because of the many current issues associated with diagnostic and treatment services on the hospital campus, specific strategies and actions should be defined to guide ongoing investments in facility upgrading and acquisition of new technology and medical equipment.

Outpatient Service Configuration and Provision of Physician Office Space

Most healthcare organizations require a focused facility investment strategy that corresponds to their market strategies for penetrating target markets and increasing market share, physician recruitment, development of centers of excellence, and so on. The facility development strategy may address construction of freestanding, community-based outpatient facilities; new outpatient facilities in partnership with surgeons or physician specialists; expansion or construction of physician office space on the hospital campus; or expansion of existing space for new or growing programs or services.

In particular, a strategy may be developed to move high-volume, routine outpatient services off site to less costly and more easily accessible facilities. This approach also reduces traffic and congestion on the main hospital campus and frees parking spaces. Examples include outpatient physical therapy, radiation oncology, dialysis, and primary care clinics.

Building Infrastructure Upgrading and Equipment Acquisition/Replacement

Unless a specific healthcare facility has been replaced within the recent decade, a strategy is generally required to address the need for continued maintenance and updating of the physical plant as facilities are retooled and renewed to meet changing demand and technology. Actions related to the acquisition or replacement of new equipment are also frequently included as part of a long-range facility investment strategy and should be integrated with the organization's IT strategic plan.

Patient Experience Improvement

In an effort to promote customer loyalty, provide a healing environment, and satisfy employers and payers, most healthcare organizations include some aspect of improving the patient's experience as one of their facility investment strategies. This may involve improving wayfinding and access to necessary services, collocating related services to provide one-stop shopping, and upgrading the interior decor and provision of enhanced amenities. I have found that an understanding of the following points is key to improving the patient's experience.

All Patients Are Not the Same

Healthcare customers tend to simply be categorized as inpatients or outpatients. Just as inpatients vary from the acutely ill with life-threatening conditions to the short-stay patient undergoing a routine procedure, outpatients also have different needs and expectations depending on their acuity and the nature of the care that they require. At the same time, the distinction between an inpatient and an outpatient is blurring with new care delivery models, alternate care settings, and technological advances. Today, unless admitted through the ED, most patients arrive at the hospital as an outpatient and are generally admitted post-procedure. With the explosion of minimally invasive surgery and same-day medical procedures, the only difference between an inpatient and an outpatient is often the length of their recovery—for example, four, six, or eight hours versus a 30-hour stay or next-day discharge. These patients experience the same reception and intake processes and require the same predischarge instructions regardless of whether they are classified as an inpatient or outpatient.

There are also different types of outpatients, as shown in Figure 6.1, ranging from those seeking care for life-threatening conditions to those focused on fitness and wellness. Various types of care for outpatients include the following:

- Emergency/urgent care that requires immediate treatment for life-threatening or urgent conditions, as well as care for patients who consider themselves to be in immediate need of medical care

- Routine/episodic care may involve an occasional or once-a-year visit to the healthcare campus for routine care, such as an annual physical or a chest x-ray

FIGURE 6.1   DIFFERENT TYPES OF OUTPATIENTS

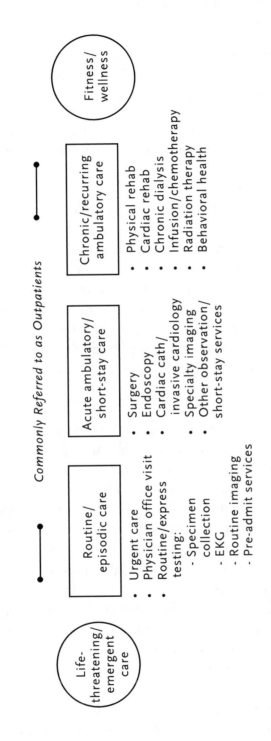

Commonly Referred to as Outpatients

Life-threatening/ emergent care

Routine/ episodic care

- Urgent care
- Physician office visit
- Routine/express testing:
  - Specimen collection
  - EKG
  - Routine imaging
  - Pre-admit services

Acute ambulatory/ short-stay care

- Surgery
- Endoscopy
- Cardiac cath/ invasive cardiology
- Specialty imaging
- Other observation/ short-stay services

Chronic/recurring ambulatory care

- Physical rehab
- Cardiac rehab
- Chronic dialysis
- Infusion/chemotherapy
- Radiation therapy
- Behavioral health

Fitness/ wellness

Source: Hayward, C. 2005. *SpaceMed—A Space Planning Guide for Healthcare Facilities.* Ann Arbor, MI: Hayward & Associates, LLC. [Online information; retrieved 7/21/05.] www.space-med.com.

- Acute ambulatory/short-stay care may involve a once-in-a-lifetime experience, such as outpatient surgery or an outpatient cardiac catheterization

- Chronic/recurring ambulatory care involves frequent or ongoing visits, multiple times per week or month, for services such as physical therapy, cancer care, and dialysis

- Fitness/wellness activities may include exercise regimens and health education for individuals who do not perceive themselves as "patients"

Each type of outpatient has different needs and expectations relative to site access and wayfinding, convenience, recognition by staff, education, and discharge instructions. The sharing of space by different types of outpatients also needs to be considered. Viewing recovering patients exercising in a cardiac rehabilitation area may be inspirational and reassuring for a patient undergoing a heart catheterization or presurgery testing for open-heart surgery. However, it may not be advisable to mix patients undergoing chemotherapy with healthy patients undergoing annual health screening procedures.

Separating Perception from Reality
Many factors affect the patient's and staff's perceptions of inadequate facilities, as shown in Figure 6.2. Understanding the actual facility issues before investing millions of dollars in renovation or new construction is important. The initial first impression is also important, which is why the hospitality industry invests so many dollars in its entrance facades and entry lobbies. Patients may also have different perceptions and expectations depending on their age, socioeconomic status, cultural diversity, education, and exposure to the media. However, the patient's perception of high-quality care may require more than contemporary, state-of-the-art facilities. Good design should also facilitate efficient processes, eliminate clutter, and create a productive work environment for care providers. Staff attitudes may ultimately affect patient satisfaction more than facilities.

Improving the Patient Experience Does Not Always Mean Higher Costs
Acute care hospitals have been traditionally organized around departments rather than around the patients' needs. In addition to the

FIGURE 6.2 PERCEPTION OF INADEQUATE FACILITIES

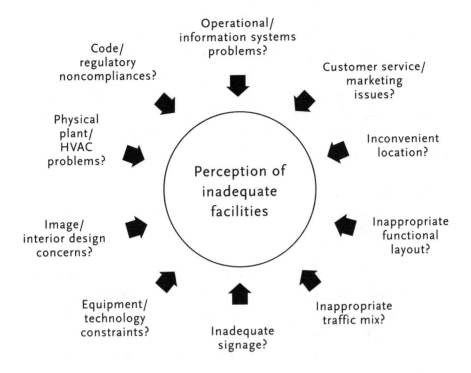

Source: Hayward, C. 2005. SpaceMed—A Space Planning Guide for Healthcare Facilities. Ann Arbor, MI: Hayward & Associates, LLC. [Online information; retrieved 7/21/05.] www.space-med.com.

customer service center and express testing concepts described in Chapter 4, other new models for delivering services to the patient result in a win-win situation by achieving both improved customer satisfaction as well as reducing costs. Examples include the following:

- Organizing patients by specialty rather than by acuity level and collocating a comprehensive range of services for a specific patient diagnosis or medical condition, such as a heart center or geriatric center;

- Creating acuity-adaptable or universal patient rooms (further described in Chapter 11); and

- Acquiring Internet-based information/communication systems that allow patients and their families access to information at any time while reducing the labor costs associated with information desks and call centers.

Improving the Patient Experience Begins Before Design
Goals to improve the patient's experience need to be established and documented well before commencement of the design process. Critical to improving the patient's experience is the integration of space programming and design with the organization's market strategy, clinical service line planning, operations redesign, and investments in new technology and information systems.

The Patient Is Not the Only Customer
For an institution to be successful, it must consider other customers and their needs:

- *Family members and visitors* may have a more extensive exposure to the organization than the patient while they are parking, waiting during the patient's procedure, and determining the patient's status at various points in time. The experience of family members and visitors may have a significant impact on the patient's perception.

- *Staff* may interact more positively with patients and their family members if they have a productive work environment and feel that they are appreciated.

- *Employers* are demanding convenient access to services, a perception by the employee of quality care, and cost-effective services for their employees.

- *Other major payers* demand cost-effective care, such as Medicare.

- *Institutional partners* may require market branding, with a consistent quality of care and facility image at all service locations.

Improving Wayfinding

Development of a simple and efficient wayfinding system to direct customers to their specific destination on the healthcare campus is closely related to any strategy for improving the patient's experience. This is becoming increasingly important in a competitive market with an aging and less ambulatory patient population. Wayfinding begins with the customer's arrival on the healthcare campus, and it involves signage and directional cues that assist the customer in identifying the appropriate building entrance, parking, and arriving at the desired service location. Key principles of wayfinding and signage for the healthcare campus include the following:

- A "shopping center" concept should be used, with an easily iden-tifiable front door supported by dedicated entrances for customers who come frequently to a specific service.

- Customers should be able to see the front door before parking their cars—everyone wants to park adjacent to the front door, so not knowing where it is creates confusion and anxiety. In particular, I have found that directional signage in parking decks, orienting the customer to the appropriate elevator and hospital entrance, is frequently overlooked in the planning of signage systems.

- The customer service center concept should be implemented and located contiguous with the main entrance, using a hub-and-spoke concept.

- A home base should be provided for families and visitors who may be arriving at different times to meet and gather, and appropriate amenities and communication systems should be available.

- Signage should serve the needs of patients and visitors; staff orientation should be done through in-service education.

- The number of potential destinations should be minimized; simple and logical names should be used for these destinations with a minimum amount of information to allow expedient decision making at any given intersection or decision node—for example, Diagnostic Center as a single destination rather than separate signs for Radiology, Nuclear Medicine, and Ultrasound.

- Signage should be consistent with constant reinforcement; this is particularly important when travel distances are lengthy. Intermittent seating should also be provided.

- Directional signage should be supplemented with architectural cues such as different floor coverings, ceiling heights, water features, statues, and dominant artwork that can be easily remembered and recalled to assist in orientation at any given point.

The development of a wayfinding program and a budget should occur in conjunction with immediate, short-term, and long-range facility reconfiguration strategies. A single administrative person should be responsible for signage and wayfinding, and a formal process should be in place for requesting new signs and for approval, ensuring consistency with the facility master plan.

Other Strategies

Depending on an organization's unique situation, additional strategies may be developed, such as the following:

- Relocate administrative offices outside the hospital to less costly and flexible space; an off-campus location may be chosen to free-up parking and reduce traffic congestion on the hospital campus.

- Relocate or consolidate selected building support services into a modernized but less costly facility; an off-campus location may be considered that can support more than one hospital site, such as a warehouse, laundry, or kitchen, or a decision may be made to outsource specific services.

- Acquire land to enlarge the current campus to replace or renew aging buildings or wings, to provide additional parking, or to construct a new physician office building or specialty center.

Figure 6.3 provides an example of a healthcare organization's key investment strategies and the corresponding actions (tasks) required for implementation of one of the strategies.

WHAT ABOUT PLANNING CENTERS OF EXCELLENCE?

Decisions to develop specific centers of excellence are complicated. An organization needs to initially understand the specific physical and virtual elements that give customers the perception of a "center" and to then identify which functional components and services will need to be physically adjacent versus virtually and electronically connected.

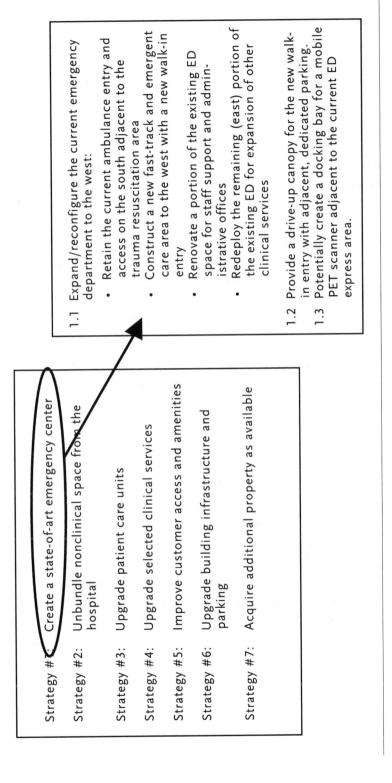

Strategy #1:   Create a state-of-art emergency center

Strategy #2:   Unbundle nonclinical space from the hospital

Strategy #3:   Upgrade patient care units

Strategy #4:   Upgrade selected clinical services

Strategy #5:   Improve customer access and amenities

Strategy #6:   Upgrade building infrastructure and parking

Strategy #7:   Acquire additional property as available

1.1   Expand/reconfigure the current emergency department to the west:

- Retain the current ambulance entry and access on the south adjacent to the trauma resuscitation area
- Construct a new fast-track and emergent care area to the west with a new walk-in entry
- Renovate a portion of the existing ED space for staff support and administrative offices
- Redeploy the remaining (east) portion of the existing ED for expansion of other clinical services

1.2   Provide a drive-up canopy for the new walk-in entry with adjacent, dedicated parking.

1.3   Potentially create a docking bay for a mobile PET scanner adjacent to the current ED express area.

Unless the center is being constructed as a freestanding facility on a new site, some physical components could be located within existing space while others are in a new addition. The trade-offs between the cost (initial capital and ongoing operational) of achieving physical adjacency versus settling for less-than-perfect convenience for the customer need to be reviewed and weighed carefully. The potential for increased revenue; reimbursement issues; and the demands of donors, partners, or investors may also affect the requirements of the physical design. Physicians often have difficulty imagining a center that is not an imposing edifice or at least a freestanding building. From the patient's perspective, once they arrive at a well-identified entrance and are greeted by a friendly and competent receptionist, they are generally oblivious to where they are treated as long as they are not asked to walk a great distance. An elevator ride with a short walk to space in an existing building is not considered a hardship, even though the physician leaders may feel that new construction is mandatory.

THE CHALLENGE OF PRIVATE DONORS

Every healthcare organization is delighted to have a private donor fund a building project. However, sometimes the donor has no interest in the organization's long-range capital investment strategy but wants to build a building or fund a program that is not even on its radar screen. Most institutions are not in a position to reject such donations, and it is a rare administrator who has the backbone to turn down money rather than to compromise the organization's long-range facility development plan. Do not be deluded into thinking there are no strings attached to donor money. These projects can become very difficult and emotionally draining. It helps, though, if the fundraising arm of the organization is integrated with the facility planning process such that the organization can seek donations that are aligned with its long-range facility master plan. Most importantly, the real issue associated with constructing an unnecessary or oversized building is affording the ongoing operational costs even though the initial construction is financed by someone else (Waite 2005).

IS "DOING NOTHING" A STRATEGY?

It is not unusual today for board members to ask the question, What happens if we do nothing? This may appear to be a viable strategy

FIGURE 6.4 EXAMPLE: FUTURE DEPARTMENT LOCATION DRAWING

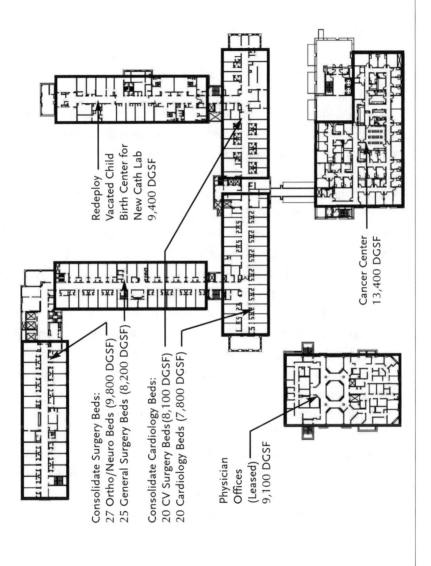

Redeploy
Vacated Child
Birth Center for
New Cath Lab
9,400 DGSF

Cancer Center
13,400 DGSF

Consolidate Surgery Beds:
27 Ortho/Neuro Beds (9,800 DGSF)
25 General Surgery Beds (8,200 DGSF)

Consolidate Cardiology Beds:
20 CV Surgery Beds(8,100 DGSF)
20 Cardiology Beds (7,800 DGSF)

Physician
Offices
(Leased)
9,100 DGSF

for an organization that is looking for a merger partner or is trying to conserve capital to build a replacement facility. However, it is important to differentiate between doing nothing and maintaining the status quo. Just to maintain the status quo, and ensure that market share does not erode and that key staff do not leave, money will need to be spent to maintain critical building systems and to upgrade furnishings and finishes to uphold a clean and professional image.

FUTURE FACILITY CONFIGURATION DRAWINGS

Once consensus has been reached on future strategies and corresponding actions, future department location drawings will need to be prepared that show the future size and location of all departments at the conclusion of the proposed renovation or reconfiguration, new construction, or demolition. They may be highlighted graphically to illustrate phasing stages over time as appropriate. A site plan may also be required that illustrates proposed changes to site access, circulation, building entry points, designated parking areas, and new additions or replacement facilities. Supplemental diagrams and graphics are frequently used as communication tools, such as the building section, or stacking, diagrams described in Chapter 2. An example of a typical future department location drawing is illustrated in Figure 6.4.

Depending on the abilities of your inhouse resources, such as your in-house architect, and whether you are using outside assistance from a predesign planning consultant, you may need to involve a design consultant at this point to perform a feasibility study, particularly if major facility expansion is anticipated. This study may include an analysis of alternative siting options, horizontal or vertical expansion trade-offs, and facility reuse issues. However, most predesign planning consultants, who specialize in facility master planning, will have licensed architects on their staff to routinely assist with the translation of your facility development strategies into facility reconfiguration actions (or options as applicable) in conjunction with strategy development.

REFERENCE

Waite, P. S. 2005. *The Non-Architect'ss Guide to Major Capital Projects: Planning, Designing, and Delivering New Buildings.* Ann Arbor, MI: Society for College and University Planning.

CHAPTER SEVEN

Identifying Specific Projects and Preparing a Phasing/Implementation Plan

O NCE CONSENSUS HAS been reached on a long-range facility investment plan, the translation of the strategies and corresponding actions into defined projects can commence. Specific projects are generally grouped and sequenced based on the following:

- Urgency, such as in response to a competitive threat, code issues, or revenue generation

- Renovation or construction feasibility and cost effectiveness

- Available capital at different points in time

- Bandwidth of the organization to handle multiple ongoing projects

The detailed phasing/implementation plan lists each project, the required sequencing, and the corresponding capital needs over time. Various types of project planning and management software are available to track each specific project's actual expected start date, completion date, and the person responsible for its oversight. Figure 7.1

Healthcare Facility Planning: Thinking Strategically

FIGURE 7.1 EXAMPLE: DETAILED PROJECT PHASING/IMPLEMENTATION PLAN

Preliminary Estimated Project Cost (in millions)

Task	Project	Pre-Task	Site	2004	2005	2006	2007	2008	2009	2010	2011	2012	2013	Total
1.1	Relocate plant operations (3M)	—	LMH	$0.30										$0.30
1.2	Consolidate home health (leased)	—	Off	tbd										$0.00
1.3	Demolish south metal building	1.1	LMH	$0.25										$0.25
1.4	Create new parking spaces	1.3	LMH	$0.15										$0.15
2.1	Convert 5N to office occupancy	—	LMH		$1.00									$1.00
2.2	Relocate IS (Jewett to 5N)	2.1	LMH	$0.10										$0.10
2.3	Relocate volunteers (Jewett to Cox)	4.5	LMH	$0.10										$0.10
2.4	Demolish Jewett wing	2.3	LMH		$0.15									$0.15
2.5	Create new parking spaces	2.4	LMH		$0.25									$0.25
3.1	Create patient service center	4.2	LMH		$1.50									$1.50
3.2	Upgrade surgery suite (2E)	3.1	LMH			$3.50								$3.50
3.3	Create ICU/CCU beds (2W)	3.2	LMH				$1.50							$1.50
3.4	Convert 7/8N to office occupancy	3.3	LMH					$1.50						$1.50
3.5	Reconfigure OP services (1st floor)	3.1	LMH			$3.25								$3.25
3.6	Convert 4M neuro unit	3.4	LMH						$4.00					$4.00
3.7	Upgrade 2M (ortho)	3.6	LMH							$0.75				$0.75
3.8	Convert 3M for oncology unit	3.6	LMH							$3.00				$3.00
3.9	Convert 6N to office occupancy	3.8	LMH								$1.60			$1.60
3.10	Demolish Cox wing/improve facade	3.9	LMH									$0.60		$0.60
4.1	Upgrade surgery/recovery	—	CCH	$0.75										$0.75
4.2	Convert 2N to generic/business office	4.1	CCH	$0.50										$0.50
4.3	Upgrade ED	—	CCH	$0.50										$0.50
4.4	Upgrade selected clinical services	—	CCH	$2.40	$1.00									$3.40
4.5	Consolidate HR (1M)	1.2	CCH		$0.50									$0.50
4.6	Consolidate laboratory	4.5	CCH		$0.50									$0.50
4.7	Upgrade 2E/W	—	CCH			$0.50								$0.50
	Total			$5.05	$4.90	$7.25	$1.50	$1.50	$4.00	$3.75	$1.60	$0.60	$0.00	$30.15

provides an example of a summary format used by a senior leadership team to communicate projects and dollars as part of the funding approval process.

GROUPING OF PROJECTS BY PRIORITY

Projects are generally grouped according to their priority as follows:

- *Immediate priority* for projects that must be completed as soon as possible (even though renovation or construction may take up to two years)

- *Short-term priority* for projects that must be completed within two to five years) and for which planning needs to be initiated promptly

- *Long-range priority* for projects where completion is anticipated to be needed beyond five years and after the immediate and short-term projects have been completed. The need for these projects would generally be reconfirmed at some point during the initial five-year time frame and may be based on achievement of critical benchmarks

- *Independent* projects should also be identified—for example, if a project's timing and completion is relatively independent from the other projects or if specific benchmarks are established that would trigger implementation (such as a census increase over multiple fiscal quarters) Certificate of Need submittal by a competitor, or donor funding

DEVELOPING PRELIMINARY PROJECT COST ESTIMATES

During the predesign planning stage, there is limited information available regarding construction conditions, the quality of construction anticipated, the construction bidding climate, and other factors that could influence the total project cost. Although it is necessary to establish an early "order of magnitude" estimate for the cost of construction or renovation, estimates made at this time should be regarded with caution. Typically, the process for developing a preliminary cost estimate includes first estimating the *base construction cost* and then applying a series of factors or additional budget items to estimate the *total project cost*.

To estimate the base cost of renovation, the anticipated cost of new construction can be factored as follows:

- *Minor renovation* includes construction with minimal demolition of existing walls and utilization of existing utilities, and it is usually 25 percent to 35 percent of the cost of new construction.

- *Moderate renovation* assumes the reuse of the primary mechanical systems, with some demolition of existing walls, and it is usually 50 percent to 60 percent of the cost of new construction.

- *Major renovation* assumes the complete demolition of the existing walls and major reworking of the mechanical systems, and it is generally around 75 percent of the cost of new construction. However, some major renovation may actually be equal to or greater than the cost of new construction.

Base construction cost estimates are calculated and totaled for all facility components to be included in the project using either DGSF, if the project includes the renovation of specific departments, or BGSF, if the project includes new construction.

Once the base construction cost is estimated, the total project cost can be estimated by budgeting additional dollars for the following:

- Site work can be estimated at 10 percent for new construction.

- Multilevel parking can be estimated based on the national average of $11,315 per space (*ENR* 2004) and 40 percent to 60 percent higher for underground parking (Rowland 2004).

- Moveable equipment, furniture, and furnishings are some of the most difficult elements to estimate during predesign planning and may vary from 10 percent to 40 percent, depending on factors such as the extent of equipment to be reused and vendor discounts. Typically, major imaging equipment is purchased separately from the construction budget, and it is therefore accounted for separately. Alternately, a single dollar figure can be budgeted or a list developed of specific major medical equipment items.

- A building and construction contingency factor of 10 percent is usually added to allow for unknown costs that cannot be identified at the start of construction.

- Project-related fees for programming consultants, architects, equipment planners, construction managers, interior designers, and so on may total 10 percent to 15 percent of the base construction cost.

- Other costs, such as the cost of land acquisition, testing and inspections, administrative and legal fees, and financing costs, should be added as appropriate.

An *inflation factor* may need to be added to adjust the base construction cost to reflect future construction conditions. Most contractors will adjust their construction estimates to the midpoint of construction to account for anticipated inflation in labor and materials if the project is large and to be constructed over a multi-year time period—for example, a 1 percent to 2 percent increase to the midpoint of construction.

DIFFERENTIATING BETWEEN BASE CONSTRUCTION COSTS AND PROJECT COSTS

After additional costs for all of the above factors are tabulated, they should be added to the base construction cost to arrive at the total project cost. Just as confusing net and gross space can lead to misunderstandings (as described in Chapter 2), confusing the base construction cost and project cost can also lead to problems. Facility planners, architects, and even construction specialists often refer to "cost" without qualifying whether it is simply the base construction cost or the total amount that must be funded (project cost). This can be disastrous, because the project cost may be 50 percent to 70 percent higher than the base construction cost.

PREPARING REALISTIC COST ESTIMATES: A CATCH-22 SITUATION

The preparation of a project cost estimate at the predesign (and schematic design) stage often presents a Catch-22 situation, where the desired outcome is difficult to attain because of inherent but well-intentioned conflicts of interest. Project cost estimates may be provided by one or more people involved in the facility planning process, including the architect, the construction manager, a professional cost estimator, the hospital-based facility manager, or a facility planning or project management consultant.

If asked to prepare the project cost estimate, an architect who may eventually be awarded the design contract may understate the complexity and cost of the project for fear that the project might be derailed or downsized and the design concept jeopardized. A construction manager who may eventually be charged with delivering the completed project on budget may provide an overly conservative estimate. Construction managers are most comfortable and confident with providing cost estimates based on a set of detailed architectural drawings and specifications, and they naturally overcompensate when only limited information concerning a potential project is available. If the project cost estimate is too high, the potential project may be deemed infeasible or the project may be literally sent "back to the drawing board." Valuable staff time and professional fees are wasted when the project is appropriate and affordable but derailed because of a conservatively high cost estimate. The same thing can happen when the project cost is understated and requires redesign midstream, resulting in expensive "change orders."

This push–pull situation can be modulated with an adept facility manager who has experience at the particular healthcare facility. A hospital-based facility manager can provide historical comparisons based on previous renovation or construction projects at the specific campus. A knowledge of unique construction conditions, the quality of construction anticipated by the organization's leadership, and the organization's corporate culture regarding decision making have a major impact on the accuracy of early predesign project cost estimates. At the predesign planning stage, professional cost estimators will have little to contribute and, like construction specialists, may be overly conservative. Input from an experienced facility planning consultant will provide objectivity and will help an organization focus on the broader question: Can the specific organization implement its immediate and short-term projects with the available capital resources? As the facility planning process progresses and an increasing amount of detail is developed, some projects will require more dollars, but others will require less such that the overall budget will be appropriate.

Ultimately, a healthcare organization should hire planning, design, and construction professionals who can assist the owner in getting the best project within a fixed budget by evaluating various trade-offs and weighing the advantages and disadvantages. This may range from decisions related to operational concepts and their impact on staffing, equipment, and space needs to evaluating alternative architectural design solutions and comparing trade-offs between the quality and the quantity of space.

PLANNING A NEW FACILITY FROM THE GROUND UP

The planning of a replacement hospital or a new freestanding health-care facility requires a different approach, because the entire facility becomes the project. Although in some cases phased construction may be planned, a master project budget is generally developed that addresses all aspects of the project from start to completion. John Kemper's (2004) book *Launching a Capital Project* provides an example of a sample master project budget that addresses the various costs associated with the planning, design, and construction of a new or replacement healthcare facility.

REFERENCES

Engineering News-Record (ENR). 2004. http://www.enr.com.

Kemper, J. 2004. *Launching a Capital Project*. Chicago: Health Administration

Rowland, J. D. 2004. "How Much Will My New Parking Structure Cost?" *The Parking Professional* (January): 13–17.

CHAPTER EIGHT

Beginning Detailed Operational and Space Programming

D ETAILED OPERATIONAL (FUNCTIONAL) and space program-ming begins once a specific project has been defined, approved, and funded. This final stage of the predesign plan-ning process generally begins once consensus has been reached on an appropriate long-range facility investment strategy and a phasing/imple-mentation plan has been prepared. Detailed operational and space pro-grams should be prepared for immediate or short-term projects for which planning needs to commence. This process provides a forum to rethink operational processes and the use of technology such that facility investments enhance operational efficiency and improve customer serv-ice, in addition to providing newer, code-compliant, and aesthetically pleasing facilities. After administrative approval, the operational and space program becomes an "approved" document serving as a control mechanism for all members of the planning and design team during the schematic drawing and design development phases of the architectural design process. The operational and space programming document should provide all necessary information for the design architect to begin schematic design.

DEFINING OPERATIONAL AND SPACE PROGRAMMING

Operational and space programming, as it is defined today, includes the two-step process of documenting the operational (functional) planning assumptions and preparing a detailed space listing (space program). Traditionally, a list of spaces and their corresponding sizes was the only written documentation preceding facility design. Today, operational planning precedes space planning, and one document—the operational and space program—combines the results of both processes. Although the terms *functional and space programming* and *functional space programming* are commonly used, I prefer to use the term *operational and space programming* throughout this book to emphasize the rigor that should be involved at this critical point in the facility planning process.

The tasks necessary to develop a detailed operational and space program are among the most critical in the facility development process. From my experience, long-term operational costs often exceed the initial capital cost of renovation and construction in a couple of years. Efficient planning at this stage will save significant operational dollars in the future. Also, paying careful attention to the development of realistic workload projections and differentiating between actual space needs versus wish lists will guard against the construction of inappropriate and inflexible space and will eliminate overbuilding.

COMPONENTS OF THE OPERATIONAL PROGRAM

The operational program should provide a description of the scope of services and operational concepts as well as the numbers and categories of people, systems, and equipment necessary to operate the specific department or service line at a projected workload level. The operational program should also address facility layout considerations, necessary and desired physical proximities, and opportunities to achieve operational flexibility and accommodate future growth. Although the outline can be tailored to meet an organization's specific situation, typical components of the operational program are described below, along with sample text that illustrates the scope and level of detail that should be provided.

EXAMPLE: OPERATIONAL PROGRAM FOR AN ENDOSCOPY SUITE

Current Situation (Baseline)

The current scope of services, space allocation, and location should be identified, and deficiencies requiring correction should be documented.

> Mercy Medical Center (MMC) currently operates two endoscopy suites. One is located on the second floor of the Ambulatory Care Center (ACC) on the MMC main campus, and the other is located on the second floor of the Mercy East Campus (MEC) hospital.
>
> - *MMC.* This suite currently has seven procedure rooms and occupies approximately 4,580 departmental square feet (DGSF). Only six rooms are used because one of the procedure rooms is small and difficult to use. The suite also has 12 patient prep/recovery bays that are undersized, and there is limited area for patient nourishments, linens, supply storage, and trash holding. There is no fluoroscopy capability within the suite, so ERCP's are done within a dedicated fluoroscopy room in the main radiology department. Bronchoscopies are performed in the pulmonary lab with nursing coverage provided by the endoscopy department.
>
> - *MEC.* This endoscopy suite is composed of five procedure rooms (four endoscopy and one bronchoscopy), occupying 4,470 DGSF. The rooms are adequately sized with contiguous patient toilet rooms. Patient prep and recovery functions occur within the shared 30-bed ambulatory recovery area on the fourth floor of the hospital.

Future Vision and Planning Goals

Strategic (market) planning and operational performance improvement goals pertaining to the specific department or service line should be specified to keep the planning team focused on the expected results.

> MMC is considering consolidation of the endoscopy suite located on the third floor of the MEC with the endoscopy suite located on the second floor of the ACC on the MMC main campus. It is anticipated that the consolidated suite will continue to be located on the second floor of the ACC. Adjacent expansion space is

potentially available because of the recently vacated dialysis unit (5,350 DGSF); other adjacent space currently used for private physician offices could also be relocated.

Other assumptions include the following:

- Outpatient registration will continue to occur on the first floor of the ACC, and patients will then proceed to the second floor endoscopy waiting area.

- Bronchoscopy procedures will be consolidated at MMC as well. These procedures will continue to be done within the pulmonary lab with nursing coverage provided by the endoscopy staff.

- ERCPs will eventually be moved to the consolidated endoscopy suite with the timing dependent on acquisition of a new digital unit. In the short-term, ERCPs will continue to occur within the main radiology department on the first floor of MMC.

Current and Projected Workloads

A detailed analysis of the current and future workloads for patient care functions can involve evaluation of case mix and scheduling patterns, as well as the interrelationship between the volume and timing of arrivals, desirable waiting times, and the number of procedure rooms or workstations. Identification of average and peak workloads is particularly important for those services whose workload is primarily a random occurrence, such as emergency visits and obstetrics deliveries.

A total of 12,096 patients received gastroscopy or bronchoscopy procedures in 2004:

- 9,222 procedures at MMC (8,853 GI procedures and 369 bronchoscopies)

- 2,874 procedures at MEC (2,759 GI procedures and 115 bronchoscopies)

Approximately 55 percent of the total procedures are colonoscopies and 30 percent are gastro procedures. In addition, flexible sigmoidoscopies, ERCP, esophageal motility, TEE, 24-hour pH monitoring, and bronchoscopies are performed. Outpatient procedures represent 90 percent of the total volume. The combined workload is projected to grow at a rate of

1 percent per year assuming that all physicians from MEC move toward consolidation at MMC.

Assuming an increase to approximately 12,200 procedures (excluding bronchoscopies) over the next five years, a total of six to seven procedure rooms, four prep/holding spaces, and 14 recovery bays are required. Seven procedure rooms have been programmed to provide the flexibility to include other procedures (e.g., bronchoscopies) in the future.

Planned Hours of Operation

Assumptions regarding the planned hours of operation by daily shift and by days of the week should be specified.

It is anticipated that the consolidated endoscopy service will operate approximately 12 hours per day, Monday through Friday, 5:30 a.m. to 5:30 p.m. Procedures will generally be scheduled between 6:00 a.m. and 3:00 p.m. as well as on Saturdays (e.g., 8:00 a.m. to 12:00 p.m.) if staff are available.

Current and Future Staffing

The numbers, categories, and work scheduling patterns of people who will be working within the department should be documented. Staffing primarily affects the provision of administrative spaces such as offices, workstations, conference rooms, and lounges. Scheduling patterns are of particular importance in determining the number of people on the day (or primary shift) for which space is planned. Most importantly, the future types and numbers of full-time equivalents (FTEs) should be reviewed relative to projected future workloads to ensure that the new or expanded facilities do not require additional staff that cannot be justified based on workload growth.

A single manager currently oversees the combined department with team leaders at both sites. There are currently 28.95 FTEs (July payroll) as follows:

- 5.25 FTEs at MEC

- 23.70 FTEs at MMC

The proposed staffing for the consolidated department is estimated at 26.30 FTEs, resulting in a reduction of 2.65 FTEs even though a 5 percent increase in workload is expected within five years.

Position	MEC FTEs	MMC FTEs	Consolidated Staffing (Day Shift)
Manager	—	1.0	1.0
Team leader	1.0	1.0	1.0
Registered Nurse	—	1.0	1.0
Specialty Registered Nurse I	0.5	3.0	3.0
Specialty Registered Nurse II	1.0	1.9	2.5
Specialty Registered Nurse III	—	4.8	4.8
GI technician	2.75	5.0	7.0
Lead GI tech specialist	—	3.0	3.0
Tech assistant I	—	1.0	1.0
Clerk receptionist	—	1.0	1.0
Surgical services assistant	—	1.0	1.0
Total	5.25	23.7	26.3

Equipment, Technology, and Support Systems

Major equipment items and support systems should be documented because of their impact on both space need and capital requirements. Equipment units that take up floor space and other items that either represent a significant capital expense or have a direct effect on productivity should be identified. The significance of equipment and support systems will vary depending on the department or service line.

Equipment at both the MEC and MMC endoscopy suites varies relative to its age and usefulness:

- *MEC.* The scopes used in the four rooms at MEC are eight years old. The department is currently evaluating a lease option for Pentax scopes based on a fee-per-procedure model. The existing equipment can be used as backup equipment.

- *MMC.* The Olympus scopes used in the six rooms at MMC are in good condition.

In summary, no additional endoscopy equipment will be required to accommodate the combined workload. The existing radiographic/fluoroscopic room in the radiology department used for ERCP's is 15 years old. Replacement of the radiographic/fluoroscopic equipment with a digital unit should be considered in the consolidated endoscopy suite.

In particular, assumptions regarding institutionwide support systems such as IT, central scheduling, and materials management should be documented and coordinated through central sources within the organization.

Preliminary operational assumptions for the consolidated endoscopy suite include the following:

- *Registration.* Patients are essentially 100 percent preregistered. Patients will complete registration and have insurance verified at the registration area on the first floor of the ACC.

- *Scheduling.* A centralized scheduling system is in place to optimize patient convenience and staff/physician workflow.

- *Cashiering.* Payments by credit card and check will be accepted at the point of service. Cash payments will be directed to the cashier in the Customer Service Center.

- *Telecommunications.* The central hospital switchboard will be used and supported by the MMC telecommunication system.

- *Information systems.* Order entry and results reporting will be fully automated using the ESI system. Patient demographics and archives will be available to support patient registration. Digital dictation will be continued in the consolidated department using the outsourced Medquest system.

- *Medical records.* The endoscopy department retrieves medical records for clinic patients on the day of the procedure. For all outpatients, the department creates a departmental record that is held for seven years on site.

- *Linen.* Linen for the endoscopy suite will continue to be provided by the same contract linen service used by MMC and delivered to the department on a routine and requisition basis. With the consolidation, additional inventory will be needed within the suite.

- *Medications.* The endoscopy suite will be supported from the MMC pharmacy. Limited stock medications (narcotics, antibiotics, antiemetics, etc.) are kept within the suite. Ideally, a Pyxis unit should be used to track medications (MEC currently uses Pyxis.)

- *Scope processing.* The endoscopy suite will continue to reprocess endoscopes. No central reprocessing of instruments at MMC, in support of the consolidated suite, is anticipated.

- *Supply storage.* Bulk supplies will be received and stored by the MMC materials management department and delivered to the endoscopy suite in retail form on a routine and requisition basis; supplies will be stocked on mobile carts.

- *Hazardous waste.* Hazardous waste will be bagged and held in the soiled utility areas until picked up by environmental services.

- *Patient transportation.* The endoscopy suite utilizes aides for transport of inpatients to and from nursing units.

- *Food.* Food service will be provided from the MMC kitchen as needed (e.g., snacks for outpatients). Staff will utilize the food court on the second floor of the hospital and a staff lounge/break room is provided within the department.

- Parking. It is assumed that sufficient parking capacity will be available at the MMC parking garage to accommodate patients/visitors. Staff will continue to park in the staff parking lot, and physicians will continue to park in the physicians' parking lot.

Functional Adjacencies and Access

For departments involved in direct patient care, patient access should be defined, including assumptions regarding site access, parking, building access points, and unique signage and wayfinding requirements. Optimal interdepartmental and intradepartmental functional adjacencies should also be noted.

> The existing reception and waiting area on the second floor, with nearby elevator access, can continue to be used, although ideally it should be reconfigured or enlarged to accommodate the additional patient volume.

> Outpatients will complete registration and check-in at the registration area on the first floor and then proceed to the second floor reception area of the consolidated suite. Outpatients will change within their prep cubicle or a changing booth. Patient lockers will be provided where changing booths are provided.

A public/staff corridor connection must be maintained on the second floor to facilitate circulation between the ACC elevators and the rest of the hospital complex (via the East and West Pavilions).

Future Trends and Operational Flexibility
Planning uncertainties as a result of future trends should be identified, and opportunities to achieve flexibility should be noted as well.

Endoscopy workload fluctuations, physician scheduling patterns, and reimbursement changes should be closely monitored to detect their potential impact on future utilization of the MMC endoscopy suite. Because outpatients represent 90 percent of the current workload, the workload could fluctuate substantially over time depending on the physicians' continued interest in performing these procedures at MMC versus in their office suites.

Outstanding Issues to Be Resolved
Issues that require additional input from senior management or physician leaders should be documented along with a time frame for resolution.

It is assumed that bronchoscopies will continue to be performed in the pulmonary lab at MMC. Additional procedure room capacity may be needed within the endoscopy suite if it is decided that these procedures will be performed within the suite. Bronchoscopy volume is projected to be approximately 500 per year (two patients per day).

Although it appears that there is adequate procedure space for consolidating the services at the MMC campus, the existing suite is extremely deficient in support space. Relocating the prep and recovery function to the vacated dialysis area (or other vacated space) and providing additional support space within the existing suite should be considered.

Although eventual relocation of the radiographic/fluoroscopic unit from the main radiology department to the endoscopy suite is planned, this move should occur at such time that the equipment is replaced with a digital unit (within two years). An additional procedure room has been programmed that can be shelled until the equipment is replaced and the decision to relocate this service to the endoscopy suite is confirmed.

Preparation of the operational program is typically an iterative process beginning with the accumulation of baseline data for the specific department or functional area to be programmed—for example, current and projected workloads, staffing, equipment, space allocation, and existing deficiencies. A listing of preliminary functional and operational assumptions can be developed for initial review by a designated task force charged with its development. The task force, or *user group*, should include department or service line leadership as well as other key stakeholders. The draft operational (functional) program narrative is refined at subsequent task force meetings (typically three meetings) and finalized. At this point, the preparation of the space program can begin.

PREPARING THE SPACE PROGRAM

Space programming is the process by which the operational program is translated into room-specific space requirements, and it can begin once the functional and operational planning assumptions are documented. The space program should provide a tabulation of every room or area required with the assigned function, number (or units), area needed for each unit to perform the function, and total area required for the function. Comments for each space should also be provided regarding the location of the space relative to other spaces, the minimum dimensions, the major equipment items to be accommodated in the space, and any special performance or environmental requirements as shown in Table 8.1.

Generally, the process begins with a list of spaces to be included for a selected department or functional area, proceeds to the preparation of a draft space program to be reviewed by the designated task force, and concludes with the approval of the space program by the task force members. Architectural design (schematic design) should only begin after task force members approve and sign-off on the operational and space program.

ORGANIZING THE SPACE PROGRAM

The space program should be organized by major category of space to facilitate review by different constituencies, such as the following:

- *Patient intake space,* including reception, registration, patient and visitor waiting, and related amenities

TABLE 8.1 EXAMPLE: DETAILED SPACE PROGRAM

Room/Area	Unit	NSF	Total NSF	Comments
Receptionist workstation	2	40	80	Locate proximate to waiting room and entrance to procedure area
Family waiting area	1	270	270	Seating for up to 18 visitors, television, coffee station, and coat rack
Interview/consult room	1	100	100	Seating for 6 to 8 people
Public toilet	1	50	50	Wheelchair accessible
Subtotal (Patient Intake Area)			500	
Patient lockers/storage	20	3	60	Purse/tote bag lockers
Patient prep/holding bays	4	80	320	Should be adjacent to recovery suite
Exam/consult room	1	120	120	
Endoscopy procedure room	6	180	1,080	
Procedure room (shelled)	1	180	180	Shelled for future use
Recovery bays	14	80	1,120	
Patient toilet room	3	30	90	
Patient toilet room	1	50	50	Wheelchair accessible
Nurse charting/work area	1	180	180	Charting station with view of recovery bays; each to include phone and computer
Medication station	1	20	20	Pyxis unit with access to sink, refrigerator, and double-locked storage
Nourishment station alcove	1	20	20	Sink, refrigerator, and ice machine
Emergency equipment alcove	1	20	20	Located within recovery suite

TABLE 8.1 (CONTINUED)

Clean supply room	1	160	160	Soiled linen and trash holding, floor sink
Soiled holding room	1	100	100	Provide space for two linen carts
Linen alcove	1	20	20	
Equipment storage	1	120	120	
Wheelchair/stretcher alcove	2	30	60	
Subtotal (Procedure Suite)			*3,720*	
File room (short-term)	1	120	120	
Laser image/processor station	1	60	60	
Tech work area	1	40	40	
Physician viewing/reading room	1	80	80	
Decontamination room	1	120	120	Provide area for Steris cleaning equipment
Scope cleaning/holding room	1	120	120	Space for service sink and cart
Housekeeping closet	1	40	40	
Subtotal (Procedure Room Support)			*580*	
Private office (manager)	1	100	100	
Office (team leader)	1	80	80	
Staff lounge/break room	1	180	180	Provide counter, sink, refrigerator, microwave, and staff lockers
Staff toilet	2	50	100	At least one must be handicap accessible
Subtotal (Staff/Administrative Space)			*460*	
Total NSF			5,260	Net square feet
Net-to-department gross factor		×	1.50	
Total DGSF			7,890	Department gross square feet

- *Patient care, diagnostic, and treatment space,* such as inpatient rooms, exam rooms, procedure rooms, and treatment bays

- *Support space,* including clean and soiled utility rooms, medication rooms, and equipment storage areas that are neither used by patients nor occupied by staff on a full-time basis

- *Staff and administrative areas,* such as administrative offices and workstations, conference rooms, and staff lounges

For example, physician leaders will want to pay close attention to the patient care spaces and procedure rooms, while central registration, scheduling, and information systems staff will want to focus on patient intake space. Facilities management staff will need to review the number of procedure rooms that need to be equipped, and hospital leadership will want to review the staffing assumptions that drive the number of offices, workstations, and conference rooms.

KEY SPACE DRIVERS

A number of factors influence the type, size, and number of spaces in a given department or functional area. Key space drivers include the following:

- *Workload composition, patient mix, and scheduling patterns* primarily affect the type, number, and sizes of procedure rooms and patient preparation and recovery spaces.

- *Equipment and technology* affect the throughput of procedure rooms, which in turn affects the need for patient intake, waiting, preparation, and recovery spaces. Electronic management of information will affect the need for record storage space and will influence the flow of patients, staff, and materials throughout the department.

- *Staffing and scheduling* affect the number of staff offices and workstations needed as well as staff support facilities such as conference rooms, lockers, lounges, and toilet facilities.

- *Codes and regulations* affect the size of patient rooms, patient toilet/shower facilities, specific procedures rooms, and other space described below.

- *The organization's mission and policies* may have a significant impact on the built environment at a healthcare center. Examples that often result in increased space allocation and construction costs include the following:

  - Decisions to invest in expansive lobbies and atriums to achieve an upscale (although sometimes ostentatious) image for the organization

  - Degree of commitment within the organization to optimize the use of expensive diagnostic and treatment equipment such as MRI, CT, and PET by promoting extended hours of operation

  - Inability to establish and enforce institutionwide space standards regarding office sizes by staff hierarchy, size and use of conference rooms, staff lounges, etc.

  - Commitment to provide enhanced amenities for patients and visitors, such as comfortable lounges; dining areas; conference and education facilities; and other retail services such as gift shops, coffee shops, and an outpatient pharmacy

  - Commitment to provide enhanced amenities for physicians and employees, such as fitness centers, education and training facilities, and daycare centers

  - Education mission of the organization that requires classrooms, student lounges, and faculty offices

  - Research mission of the organization that requires space for clinical trials, offices for researchers, and dry and wet lab space

ABOUT BUILDING CODES

The space program must comply with applicable building codes. The following codes vary by state or local municipality and should be reviewed and incorporated into the final space program:

- State hospital licensing rules

- State health agency codes

- State and local building codes

- State and local fire codes

- State and local handicap accessibility standards

Many building codes specify minimum sizes for traditional inpatient rooms, procedure rooms, and other related patient care spaces (AIA and FGI 2001). The primary intent is to ensure public safety during the treatment or procedure, expedite egress for nonambulatory patients in case of a fire or other disasters, and provide accessibility for handicapped patients. Some examples of spaces for which minimum sizes are generally mandated include ED treatment cubicles, exam rooms, surgical operating rooms, labor and delivery rooms, recovery cubicles, patient toilet rooms, and private and multiple-bed inpatient rooms. The actual design and configuration of a specific room—for example, the direction of door swing or the length and width of room—and the equipment and furnishings may require minor adjustments to the space program during the design development stage.

DEVELOPING SUPPLEMENTARY CONCEPTUAL DIAGRAMS

The operational and space program will often contain supplemental "bubble" diagrams that may be drawn to scale or may simply be conceptual in nature. The intent is to illustrate department workflow, physical space proximities and adjacencies, and other concepts to educate the task force members and to communicate the intent of the operational and space program to the design architect. Figure 8.1 presents an example of a conceptual diagram that may accompany the operational and space program.

ENSURING AN EFFECTIVE PLANNING PROCESS

Historically, facility planning was often based on the wish lists of physicians and department managers. Unfortunately, some of the individuals who dominate the planning process move on to other organizations by the time the new or expanded facilities are ready for occupancy. Today, healthcare organizations realize that investments in facility expansion

FIGURE 8.1   EXAMPLE: CONCEPTUAL DIAGRAM FOR AN EMERGENCY DEPARTMENT

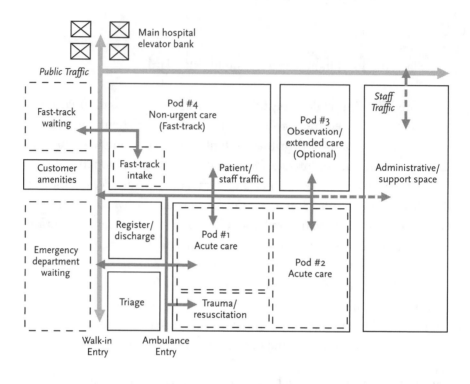

and reconfiguration must meet the needs of changing patient populations and providers during the life of the building. They cannot allow the planning process to be driven by the idiosyncrasies of a few individuals. Some healthcare organizations are challenging the more traditional bottom-up approach to operational and space planning and are choosing to embark on a more top-down approach as shown in Figure 8.2 (Hayward 2004).

Bottom-Up Approach

The traditional bottom-up approach involves the establishment of department user groups based on strict adherence to the organization's existing organizational structure. For the traditional bottom-up approach to be successful, healthcare organizations must do the following:

FIGURE 8.2 OPERATIONAL AND SPACE PROGRAMMING APPROACHES

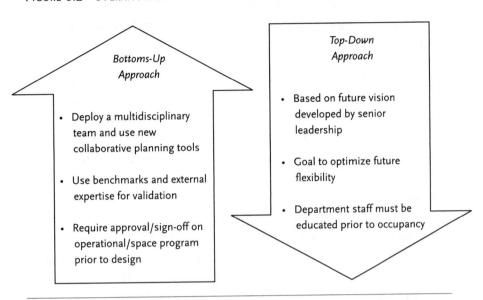

Bottoms-Up Approach

- Deploy a multidisciplinary team and use new collaborative planning tools
- Use benchmarks and external expertise for validation
- Require approval/sign-off on operational/space program prior to design

Top-Down Approach

- Based on future vision developed by senior leadership
- Goal to optimize future flexibility
- Department staff must be educated prior to occupancy

- Deploy a multidisciplinary team or task force to encourage department staff to think outside of their individual silos. Cross-departmental task forces, focused on common operational processes and patient needs, facilitate the planning of flexible healthcare space.

- Prevent specific individuals from dominating the operational and space planning process.

- Use some of the new collaborative planning tools to facilitate the gathering of input and the review of preliminary outputs. This allows multiple constituencies to participate in the process—for example, construct a project web site that can accommodate online publishing of draft documents, a 24/7 review at the participant's convenience, and easy integration of their comments.

- Use industry benchmarks and external consulting expertise to validate internally generated space requirements and to introduce the planning team to new concepts and best practices in the industry.

- Consider site visits by selected task force members to peer institutions that have implemented unique operational models or have incorporated new technology as part of their facility planning efforts.

- Require approval of the operational and space program prior to commencing the schematic design stage. A formal process should be established for use by facility management and the design architect when changes are proposed to the space program during the schematic design and design development phases.

Top-Down Approach

Some healthcare organizations prefer a more top-down approach, particularly when capital dollars are tight, when employee turnover at the department or service-line manager level is high, or when market dynamics make program and workload forecasts difficult to discern. This approach is often used when a new or replacement healthcare facility is being constructed, particularly when the leadership team wants to implement entirely new and innovative operational processes and technology. For this approach to be successful, healthcare organizations must do the following:

- Have a senior leadership team with a well-thought-out vision for the organization that can be communicated effectively.

- Bring in outside expertise to translate a future vision for the organization into flexible facilities that can accommodate future changes in medical practice and technology, accommodate various patient populations and providers, and facilitate quality and cost-effective patient care.

- Educate department staff about the vision and the new operational concepts and technology to be implemented prior to occupancy.

PROGRAMMING INPATIENT NURSING UNITS

The planning of a large number of new or replacement beds requires a significant effort if you want to end up with an operationally efficient, patient-friendly, and state-of-the-art facility. Of course, you can simply replicate your current operational concepts, level of technology, and staffing patterns with larger, newly furnished, private patient rooms. The operational and space programming process for constructing or replacing inpatient nursing units becomes somewhat more complicated than for most other hospital departments because of the magnitude of the impact of your decisions, such as labor costs and square feet. Table 8.2 summarizes the many operational issues to be resolved when planning new inpatient nursing units. Resolving these issues generally requires a larger number of participants (or more task forces). Also, all task force members must be informed and educated about current best practices and have the opportunity to make site visits to newly opened facilities and talk to their staff.

RELATIONSHIP OF THE OPERATIONAL AND SPACE PROGRAM TO SUBSEQUENT DOCUMENTATION

The operational and space program should be coordinated with the equipment procurement plan and should be reviewed by appropriate central sources such as IT, materials management, admitting and registration, and other support departments. The workload projections and staffing assumptions can be incorporated into a financial feasibility analysis.

As the design architect proceeds with the design development phase (after approval of the schematic drawings), he or she will prepare *room data sheets* that correspond to each space delineated on the drawing and include detailed design information for each space, such as floor and wall finishes; plumbing, electrical, and medical gas requirements; and similar information to be incorporated into the detailed construction documents.

When a department or service undergoes major expansion or reconfiguration or is relocated to new space, the operational and space program can provide the basis for subsequent development of an occupancy or building commissioning plan. Detailed occupancy planning generally begins as completion of the new facility approaches, and it includes items such as descriptions of new policies and procedures; revised job descriptions (as required); and a detailed schedule of tasks, dates, and responsibilities to ensure a smooth operational transition from the existing space to the new space. Because of the extended time

TABLE 8.2 SUMMARY OF NURSING UNIT OPERATIONAL ISSUES

Category	Operational Issues	Category	Operational Issues
Patient/ visitor flow	• Parking/wayfinding • Reception/information • Patient transport	Patient/ visitor flow amenities	• Television/VCR/music • PC (Internet access, video games, etc.) • Educational video (live, recorded) • Lounge/sleeping facilities • Consult/viewing
Patient processing	• Admitting • Patient transport (ancillary services, intra-unit transfers) • Discharge (home, alternate facility) • Consults (social services, pastoral care, infection control, etc.)	Clinical support	• Specimen collection/disposition/testing (e.g., point of care) • Pharmaceutical delivery/dispensing (e.g., Pyxis) • Respiratory therapy (equipment monitoring/prep/cleaning) • Physical/occupational/speech therapy • Imaging
Communications	• Telephone (conventional, wireless) • PC (intranet/Internet) • Nurse call/code blue • Electronic tracking (staff, equipment, patients, visitors) • Paging (overhead public address system, pocket pagers)	Network infrastructure	• Health information system (HIS) • Vital signs monitoring • Picture archiving communication system (PACS) • Video on demand • Telemedicine (consultative, diagnostic, LAN, WAN, etc.)
Clinical documentation	• Order entry • Results reporting • Consults • Patient demographics • Special forms • Medication profile/IV logs • Input/output • Pain management • Progress notes	Materials management	• Materials/supply distribution (barcoding, scanning) • Food delivery (conventional, cook-freeze, cook-chill, convenience) • Linen • Housekeeping • Maintenance/engineering/biomed • Patient equipment/instrument processing • Mail handling • Trash/hazardous waste
Security	• Access control • Surveillance • Detection • Disaster planning/response (security, fire, seismic, bioterrorism)		

frame from the preparation of the operational and space program through the design process to project construction and occupancy, the occupancy plan is generally developed separate from the predesign planning process and at a later date.

TEN COMMON OPERATIONAL AND SPACE PROGRAMMING PITFALLS

An understanding of the predesign planning stage, terminology, and implementation of a formal operational and space programming process will prevent most healthcare organizations from succumbing to the following top ten space planning pitfalls:

1. *Confusing net and gross space.* Department gross square feet may be 25 percent to 50 percent higher than NSF, and the BGSF may be another 25 percent to 35 percent higher than the DGSF.

2. *Planning additional procedure rooms, equipment, and expansion space for overly optimistic workload growth.* Because clinical departments typically staff based on the number of procedure rooms, deploying a "build it and they will come" approach will result in increased labor and utility costs as well as up-front equipment costs.

3. *Planning offices and workstations for future staff who have not been approved or for positions that will be eliminated.* This will create pockets of vacant or underutilized space throughout the facility; however, the creation of flexible, generic office suites for use by multiple departments can mitigate this problem somewhat.

4. *Tailoring new facilities to the idiosyncrasies of a specific department manager or physician.* Current leadership may not be around when the new facility is opened, and the replacement leadership may want to instigate a new cycle of renovation projects.

5. *Failing to consider the staffing and other operational costs associated with larger, expanded facilities.* This can be particularly problematic when revenues are flat.

6. *Replicating current, inefficient operational systems in new space.* It is more beneficial to rethink how patient care is delivered, evaluate

ways to improve customer satisfaction, and identify opportunities to provide flexible, multiuse space.

7. *Focusing on space planning and the layout while ignoring the effect of interior design, furnishings, and cosmetic improvements.* Adequate dollars must be budgeted to enhance the look and feel of the space in addition to rectifying code noncompliances and resolving space deficiencies.

8. *Neglecting to consider the impact of new medical equipment and IT on procedure room throughput and required physical proximities.* Not considering these effects will result in overbuilding as well as increased operational costs and inefficient department layouts.

9. *Not planning for less efficient space utilization when retrofitting existing space for a new function.* This will result in inappropriate and inadequate space for the planned functions. Older buildings are typically less flexible and have more unassignable space such as mechanical chases, numerous load-bearing walls and partitions that can only be removed with great difficulty and at great expense, and fixed bay widths and column spacing.

10. *Beginning schematic drawings before an approved operational and space program is completed.* Failing to wait for the completed program will result in "scope creep," with the eventual size and cost of the project potentially escalating out of control.

REFERENCES

American Institute of Architects (AIA) and Facilities Guidelines Institute (FGI). 2001. *Guidelines for Design and Construction of Health Care Facilities.* Washington, DC: American Institute of Architects Press.

Hayward, C. 2004. "Rethinking Space Programming: Process, Approach, and Tools." Paper presented at the National Symposium on Healthcare Design, Las Vegas, Nevada.

CHAPTER NINE

Developing a Ten-Year Capital Investment Strategy for a Multihospital System: A Case Study

L EE MEMORIAL HEALTH System[1] (LMHS) is the largest community-owned healthcare system in southwest Florida and is the largest, public, not-for-profit system in the state that receives no direct tax support. It is governed by a publicly elected 10-member board of directors and has served the citizens of Lee County and the surrounding communities since 1916. This progressive, financially sound healthcare provider has more than 6,700 employees, 830 physicians on staff, and 928 licensed beds. Its three acute care campuses include the following:

- *Lee Memorial Hospital (LMH),* founded in 1916, is located about a mile south of downtown Ft. Myers along a major north-south access road in the midst of a struggling commercial district. Its urban campus includes a 427-bed hospital and a medical office center that houses physicians' offices and the Rehabilitation Hospital, which has 60 inpatient beds and occupies the fifth and sixth floors. Numerous medical/surgical specialty services are provided, including a Level II trauma center.

- *HealthPark Medical Center (HPMC)* opened in 1991 to serve the growing and affluent market south of Ft. Myers and north of Naples, and it was designed with 220 beds. During the planning stage, a decision was made to relocate the cardiac surgery program from LMH to this new healthcare center and to also offer high-risk obstetrics. The Children's Hospital of Southwest Florida operates 30 beds on the second floor of HPMC, including a pediatric ICU, 40 neonatal intensive care beds (27 Level II and 13 Level III), a dedicated pediatric ED, and a range of pediatric outpatient services.

- *Cape Coral Hospital (CCH)* opened in 1977. It has served the residents of Lee County, including the communities of Cape Coral, North Ft. Myers, and Pine Island for almost 30 years and is located across a waterway with access by toll bridge. The Cape Coral community is younger, less affluent, and somewhat isolated because of its geography. Initially constructed with 94 beds, CCH has grown to its present 281 beds and provides general medical/surgical and specialty services, including high-risk obstetrics. It was acquired by LMHS in 1996 and maintains a separate medical staff.

All three hospitals have been consistently rated among the top 100 hospitals across the United States (Solucient 2005), and LMHS has received awards for its cardiac, orthopedic, and stroke programs. For several decades, it has strived to be the best patient-centered healthcare system in the state of Florida. Figure 9.1 illustrates the relative location and key characteristics of the three acute care campuses.

1999 CAPITAL INVESTMENT STRATEGY (FACILITY MASTER PLAN)

A comprehensive strategic planning process was conducted in late 1998 that identified the need for $155 million in capital investment across the three campuses, including $55 million for IT. In addition, the health system was also considering a $22 million expansion project for the Children's Hospital of Southwest Florida on the HPMC site and an investment in a "medical mall" to be located across the street.

FIGURE 9.1 LMHS's EXISTING HOSPITAL SITES AND CHARACTERISTICS

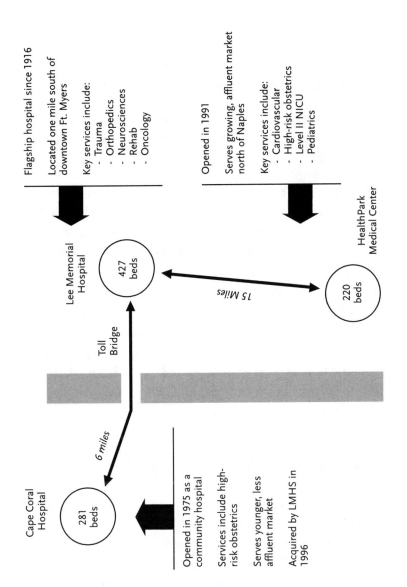

Source: Reprinted with permission from Lee Memorial Health System, Ft. Myers, Florida.

By 1999, the health system faced a number of major issues, including the following:

- *Diminishing operating margins.* Like many hospitals across the United States, LMHS's operating margins had been declining.

- *Acute nursing shortage.* The region had an acute shortage of nursing staff, particularly during the peak winter season when premium wages are paid to traveling nurses.

- *Fluctuating market dynamics.* There was concern that LMHS's high market share could diminish over time as new competitors focused on its growing market.

- *Licensed bed complement that did not reflect operational reality.* Compared to 928 total licensed beds, significantly less beds were needed even during the peak winter season. Even considering the most optimistic (high-bed) scenario, LMHS determined that it still would have a surplus of beds at the end of the decade. However, a significant portion of the licensed beds were at LMH, which was plagued by aging inpatient nursing units and lacked a sufficient number of private rooms and adequate support space to actually operate at the licensed capacity. At the same time, HPMC was at capacity and was concerned about its ability to accommodate current and future demand in its rapidly growing market.

- *Aging facilities at the flagship facility.* Almost half of LMHS's licensed beds were located at LMH, where two-thirds of the total space was constructed prior to 1970. Moreover, ongoing capital investment had been minimal over the past decade. LMH was currently staffing 324 beds during its peak winter season. However, deployment of all of its 427 licensed beds was not possible. If all 427 beds were staffed, only 37 percent of the beds would be in private patient rooms, and 17 percent of the beds would need to be placed in three-bed and four-bed wards. In contrast, the 25-year old CCH had been consistently maintained and upgraded, and the HPMC facility was just over 10 years old. Both the CCH and HPMC facilities were designed with only private patient rooms.

The LMHS decided that it needed a comprehensive facility master plan to guide capital investment over the ten-year period from 2000 to 2010. The organization also wanted to reevaluate the alignment of key clinical services among its three acute care campuses.

THE PLANNING PROCESS

The facility planning process included a review of historical utilization and market dynamics, identification of current facility assets and liabilities at the three acute care campuses, and an assessment of current and future space need by department and service line. Future bed need and ancillary workloads were forecasted, and a ten year capital investment strategy for the health system was developed. Individual interviews were conducted with department and service-line leadership, and extensive input was solicited from the physician executive committee and other physicians through individual interviews and focus group meetings. Periodic progress reports were made to the LMHS executive council and the board.

MAJOR FACILITY ASSETS AND LIABILITIES BY CAMPUS

An assessment of each campus resulted in an inventory of the facility assets and liabilities as shown in Table 9.1.

Key conclusions included the following:

- Both the LMH and CCH facilities were underutilized.

- Although HPMC was at capacity, physician offices occupied over 50,000 DGSF throughout the hospital that could be made available for other patient services if a new medical office building were constructed.

- Expansion of HPMC would require additional investment in the energy plant to increase its capacity.

- LMH has an aging physical plant that will require significant capital investment over time just to maintain the status quo.

TABLE 9.1 LMHS's MAJOR FACILITY ASSETS AND LIABILITIES BY CAMPUS

Campus	Major Facility Assets	Major Facility Liabilities
Lee Memorial Hospital (LMH)	• Located in the center of the community one mile south of downtown Ft. Myers • Level II trauma center designation • 60-bed Rehabilitation Hospital • Contiguous physician office building • On-site wellness center • Significant amount of vacant space available	• Site, parking, and wayfinding issues • Outpatient services are fragmented • General lack of public spaces and amenities • Majority of medical/surgical beds are in older wings with limited private rooms and some older wards • Seperation of the medical/surgical ICUs create staffing inefficiencies and limits flexibility • Cox/Jewett wings have severe code deficiencies
HealthPark Medical Center (HPMC)	• Newer facility with a high-level of aesthetic appeal (e.g., large atrium) • All inpatient beds in contemporary, private rooms • Ample land for facility expansion • High-profile cardiovascular service • High-profile NICU/obstetrics service with 36 LDRPs • The Children's Hospital offers specialty pediatric services • Contiguous physician office space	• Outpatient services are fragmented • Multiple building entrances and intake points create further confusion • Separation of surgical services on two different floors creates operational inefficiencies • Energy plant will require upgrading to accommodate additional building expansion
Cape Coral Hospital (CCH)	• Attached Women and Children's Pavilion with dedicated entrance and 23 LDRPs • All inpatient beds in updated, private rooms • Expansion space for surgery • Contiguous physician office space • Physical plant in excellent condition • Vacant space available	• Multiple outpatient service locations with extensive walking distances, particularly from north to south • Outpatient surgery prep/recovery area requires upgrading

Source: Reprinted with permission from Lee Memorial Health System, Ft. Myers, Florida.

TABLE 9.2   LMHS'S 1999 BED COMPLEMENT

	LMH	HPMC	CCH	Total
Intensive care beds	34	23	22	79
Acute care beds	215	91	158	464
Subtotal acute beds (staffed)	249	114	180	543
Rehab beds	60			60
LDRP beds		36	23	59
Pediatric beds		30	9	39
NICU bassinets		40		40
Subtotal specialty beds (staffed)	309	220	212	741
Vacant beds	118		69	187
Current licensed beds	427	220	281	928

Source: Reprinted with permission from Lee Memorial Health System, Ft. Myers, Florida.

MARKET DYNAMICS AND FUTURE BED NEED

In aggregate, LMHS serves an older but growing population. Its service area population is expected to grow by 20 percent through 2010, with 25 percent of the population being over 65 years of age. Although the highest growth rate is occurring in south Lee County, HPMC's primary market, the highest growth in absolute numbers is occurring in Cape Coral. The consensus was that LMHS must protect its southern flank relative to cardiovascular surgery and general medical/surgical services. It was also agreed that the major competitive threat to obstetrics services will come from the east.

Table 9.2 summarizes LMHS's bed complement in 1999. A detailed bed-need analysis indicated that LMHS needed approximately 500 acute medical/surgical beds (including the ICU) during its peak winter season and about 320 beds during the summer compared to the 543 beds that are typically staffed. Use rates for Lee County were starting to decline, resulting in lower patient days despite a growing population. However, the health system consistently maintains an unusually high market share of about 67 percent.

The planning team projected that by 2010 LMHS will still have a surplus of about 150 beds compared to the current licensed capacity, even in the high-bed scenario, despite the significant population growth in Lee County. Because of fluctuating market dynamics and uncertainties, LMHS leadership was reluctant to de-license beds at the time, particularly given the substantial growth to the south. Also, because Cape Coral serves a distinct market from Ft. Myers, it was agreed that surplus beds at CCH should not be de-licensed until future population projections become evident.

KEY FACILITY PRIORITIES

Several key facility investment priorities were identified that required action regardless of LMHS's long-range facility investment strategy. These included the following:

Lee Memorial Hospital
- Reconfigure customer intake and outpatient services on the first floor to improve wayfinding, access, and convenience.

- Upgrade the surgery suite and invest in new equipment and technology to create a state-of-the-art facility.

- Combine the existing medical ICU (currently on the seventh floor) and the existing surgical ICU (currently on the eighth floor) to be on the second floor near the surgery suite to reduce staffing costs and enhance operational flexibility.

- Relocate the administrative services currently in the older Cox and Jewitt wings to the seventh and eighth floors to allow for their demolition, thus avoiding further costly maintenance of these non-code-compliant wings.

HealthPark Medical Center
- Create an express testing area adjacent to the main entry in the space to be vacated by the community pediatric clinic.

- Immediately add unlicensed short-stay and observation beds to provide additional capacity—for example, an ED holding unit, pediatric observation unit, and adult short-stay beds.

- Expand or reconfigure surgical services and add an MRI unit.

Cape Coral Hospital
- Upgrade the ED and selected clinical services (noninvasive cardiology, sleep lab, and outpatient surgery recovery area).

- Convert a portion of the second floor to administrative offices and clinical support space.

LONG-RANGE FACILITY DEVELOPMENT SCENARIOS

Three preliminary long-range facility development scenarios for the health system were identified and evaluated as follows.

Scenario 1: Maintain the Status Quo

This scenario maintains the current distribution of beds and services between the three hospital campuses and assumes the conversion of three floors of LMHS's north wing (no longer needed for inpatient space) to administrative services. The remaining five nursing units at LMH would be upgraded, and the number of private patient rooms would be increased.

Scenario 2: Decompress HPMC

The intent of this scenario was to capitalize on the underutilized Women's and Children's Pavilion at CCH by relocating high-risk obstetrics and the Children's Hospital from HPMC to CCH. In this scenario, low-risk obstetrics would remain at HPMC, and the space occupied by pediatric services and the neonatal ICU would be redeployed for additional medical/surgical bed capacity and the expanding cardiology program. The neonatal ICU would be expanded at CCH, the underutilized second-floor nursing units would be redeployed for pediatrics, and physician offices on the first floor would be reassigned for obstetricians and pediatricians.

Scenario 3: Decompress LMH

In this scenario, LMH would become a specialty center focused on orthopedics, neurosciences, and rehabilitation and would continue to maintain its trauma-center status. Its bed complement would be reduced from the licensed capacity of 427 beds to approximately 172 beds (20 ICU, 72 acute care, 20 short stay, and 60 rehabilitation). By substantially reducing its bed capacity, significant dollars would be saved that had previously been slated for upgrading its nine existing nursing units. The conversion of vacant inpatient space at LMH to office occupancy would allow the health system to consolidate various administrative services at LMH and discontinue the leasing of office space around the community.

TEN-YEAR CAPITAL INVESTMENT STRATEGY FOR LMHS

The LMHS executive council concluded that Scenario 1 was not feasible, because capital dollars were not available to maintain LMH at its current licensed bed capacity given the amount of renovation (and space) required to provide contemporary accommodations for 427 inpatients; this would be difficult even at its current staffed capacity of 324 beds. At the same time, HPMC's inpatient census continued to rise, and there was concern that LMHS was not positioned to aggressively compete for its share of the growing market south of Ft. Myers and north of Naples (one of the fastest growing areas in the United States).

Everyone agreed that CCH had surplus capacity that could be readily used for obstetric and pediatric services—HPMC had 36 LDRP rooms and exceeded 3,000 annual births while CCH had 23 LDRP rooms and ample support space with only 900 annual births. However, getting the high-risk obstetricians and pediatric specialists to move their practices from HPMC to CCH was not likely, at least not in the near future.

The executive council ultimately decided to pursue a variation of Scenario 3 that involved the transfer of 122 beds to HPMC by moving 81 medical/surgical beds from LMH and 41 beds from CCH. Specific strategies, related actions, bed allocation, and capital needs were identified over the ten-year period from 2000 to 2010, as illustrated in Figure 9.2 and described in Table 9.3.

DETAILED PROJECT PHASING/IMPLEMENTATION PLAN

LMHS's ten-year capital investment strategy was translated into distinct projects for which costs were estimated and time frames assigned, as shown in Figure 9.3. The ten-year capital investment plan for LMHS will require approximately $69 million, excluding the cost of major equipment and IT, and will be allocated as follows:

- $19 million for immediate projects to be completed within two years

- $38 million for short-term projects to be completed within three to five years

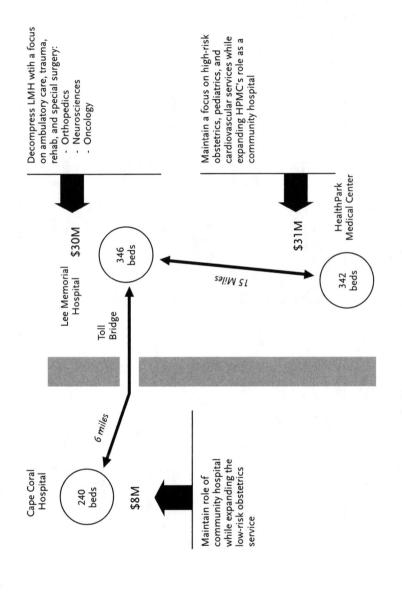

Source: Reprinted with permission from Lee Memorial Health System, Ft. Myers, Florida.

TABLE 9.3 SUMMARY OF LMHS's TEN-YEAR CAPITAL INVESTMENT STRATEGY (2000–2010)

Campus	Immediate Strategy (Within Two Years)	Short-Term Strategy (Three to Five Years)	Long-Range Strategy (Five to Ten Years)
Lee Memorial Hospital (LMH)	To improve patient intake/access and wayfinding and to demolish oldest buildings: • Create Patient Service Center • Improve patient wayfinding and signage • Demolish Jewett wing • Add patient/visitor parking spaces • Other general upgrading	Consolidate the medical and surgical ICUs, continue reconfiguring first and second floor clinical services, and convert surplus bed capacity to office occupancy: • Upgrade the surgery suite • Create consolidated ICU • Reconfigure outpatient services (first floor) • Convert 5/7/8-North to offices • Other general upgrading	Decompress LMH with a focus on ambulatory care, trauma, rehab, and special surgery: • Convert 4-MOC to neuro unit • Upgrade ortho unit • Convert 3-MOC to oncology unit • Convert 6-North to offices • Demolish Cox wing • Other general upgrading
HealthPark Medical Center (HPMC)	Address ED/bed capacity issues with specialty observation/short-stay units, and redirect low-risk obstetrics to CCH: • Create peds observation unit • Create outpatient procedure unit • Create short-stay unit • Expand the ED • Other general upgrading	Expand diagnostic/treatment services, improve outpatient intake/express testing, and increase medical/surgical bed capacity as census increases: • Convert clinic to express testing • Expand/reconfigure surgery suite • Upgrade Energy Plant • Add three floors (72-108 beds) • Add patient/visitor parking spaces • Other general upgrading	Maintain focus on high-risk obstetrics, pediatrics, and cardiovascular services while expanding HPMC's role as a community hospital

| Cape Coral Hospital (CCH) | Create office/staging space on 2-North and upgrade clinical services:
• Upgrade surgery post-op
• Convert 2-North to generic offices
• Upgrade the ED/other services
• Other general upgrading | Consolidate the clinical laboratory and upgrade/redeploy beds on second floor as census increases:
• Upgrade 2-East/West
• Consolidate laboratory
• Other general upgrading | Maintain role as a community hospital while expanding the low-risk obstetric service. |

Source: Reprinted with permission from Lee Memorial Health System, Ft. Myers, Florida.

FIGURE 9.3 LMHS's Ten-Year Project Phasing/Implementation Plan (2000–2010)

Preliminary Estimated Project Cost (in millions)

Task	Project	Pre-Task	Site	2000	2001	2002	2003	2004	2005	2006	2007	2008	2009	Total
1.1	Relocate plant operations (3M)	—	LMH	$0.30										$0.30
1.2	Consolidate home health (leased)	—	Off	tbd										$0.00
1.3	Demolish south metal building	1.1	LMH	$0.25										$0.25
1.4	Create new parking spaces	1.3	LMH	$0.15										$0.15
2.1	Convert 5N to office occupancy	—	LMH		$1.00									$1.00
2.2	Relocate IS (Jewett to 5N)	2.1	LMH	$0.10										$0.10
2.3	Relocate volunteers (Jewett to Cox)	4.5	LMH	$0.10										$0.10
2.4	Demolish Jewett wing	2.3	LMH		$0.15									$0.15
2.5	Create new parking spaces	2.4	LMH		$0.25									$0.25
3.1	Create patient service center	4.2	LMH		$1.50									$1.50
3.2	Upgrade surgery suite (2E)	3.1	LMH			$3.00								$3.00
3.3	Create ICU/CCU beds (2W)	3.2	LMH				$1.50							$1.50
3.4	Convert 7/8N to office occupancy	3.3	LMH					$2.00						$2.00
3.5	Reconfigure OP services (1st floor)	3.1	LMH			$2.50								$2.50
3.6	Convert 4M neuro unit	3.4	LMH						$4.00					$4.00
3.7	Upgrade 2M (ortho)	3.6	LMH							$0.75				$0.75
3.8	Convert 3M for oncology unit	3.6	LMH							$4.00				$4.00
3.9	Convert 6N to office occupancy	3.8	LMH						$1.00					$1.00
3.10	Demolish Cox wing/improve facade	3.9	LMH								$0.50	$0.50		$1.00
4.1	Upgrade surgery/recovery	—	CCH	$0.75										$0.75
4.2	Convert 2N to generic/business office	4.1	CCH	$1.00										$1.00
4.3	Upgrade ED	—	CCH	$0.50										$0.50
4.4	Upgrade selected clinical services	—	CCH	$1.00	$1.00									$2.00
4.5	Consolidate HR (1M)	1.2	CCH		$0.50									$0.50
4.6	Consolidate laboratory	4.5	CCH		$0.50									$0.50
4.7	Upgrade 2E/W	—	CCH			$0.50								$0.50

#	Project	Priority	Facility	$0.60/...										Total
5.1	Create peds observation unit	—	HPMC	$0.60										$0.60
5.2	Create OP procedure unit	—	HPMC	$0.20										$0.20
5.3	Create short-stay unit (17 beds)	MD	HPMC		$1.80									$1.80
5.4	Create perinatal unit (8 beds)	MD	HPMC		$1.20									$1.20
5.5	Expand ED	—	HPMC		$2.50									$2.50
5.6	Convert CMS to clinical services	MD	HPMC			$1.60								$1.60
5.7	Expand/reconfigure surgery suite	—	HPMC			$2.00								$2.00
5.8	Expand diagnostic services	—	HPMC			$1.00								$1.00
5.9	Upgrade power plant	—	HPMC			$1.00								$1.00
5.10	Add three floors (72-108 beds)	5.9	HPMC				$8.00	$8.00						$16.00
5.11	Add parking spaces/site work	—	HPMC			$1.10								$1.10
6.1	Other general upgrading	—	LMH	$1.00	$1.00	$1.00	$1.00	$1.00			$0.50	$0.50	$0.50	$5.50
6.2	Other general upgrading	—	HPMC	$0.50	$0.50	$0.50	$0.50	$0.50						$2.50
6.3	Other general upgrading	—	CCH	$0.50	$0.50	$0.50	$0.50	$0.50					$0.50	$3.00
	Total			$6.95	$11.90	$14.70	$11.50	$12.00	$5.00	$4.75	$0.50	$0.50	$1.50	$69.30

Source: Reprinted with permission from Lee Memorial Health System, Ft. Myers, Florida.

- $12 million for long-term projects to be completed beyond
  five years

UPDATE TO THE LMHS STRATEGY IN 2002

From 1999 to 2002, Lee County's population continued to grow, and the average length of stay at LMHS's facilities leveled off while its market share remained high. This resulted in improved financial performance for the health system as the census at all three campuses increased. At the same time, a significant initiative was launched by the Ft. Myers Economic Development Office to rejuvenate the downtown area and the commercial district surrounding the LMH campus. Because of these changes, LMHS leadership decided to revisit the capital investment strategy for LMH in 2002.

Lee Memorial Hospital's Functional Layout

As shown in the building section diagram in Figure 9.4, the majority of the inpatient beds at LMH are located in the older north wing. The ED and diagnostic services are located on the first floor, and the surgery suite is on the second floor. The newer Medical Office Center (MOC) is a multiuse building that houses the kitchen, laboratory, and pharmacy on the first floor and hospital administrative offices and building support services on the third and fourth floors. The inpatient orthopedics unit is located on the second floor, and inpatient rehabilitation beds (the Rehabilitation Hospital) are located on the fifth and sixth floors. Physician offices are located on the seventh and eighth floors. The third and fourth floors of the MOC could be converted to inpatient units, because the bay spacing and utility configuration is similar to that of the inpatient floors below and above.

Of LMH's 427 licensed beds, 54 percent are located in the older north wing. In particular, the medical/surgical units on the seventh and eighth floors have been closed, and the remote location of the remaining ICU beds creates significant operational inefficiencies. The Cox and Jewett wings are in severe physical disrepair and are slated for demolition as soon as the services that they house can be relocated.

Review of the Previous Facility Master Plan for LMH
Key actions identified for LMH in the 1999 facility master plan included

Source: Reprinted with permission from Lee Memorial Health System, Ft. Myers, Florida.

enhancing the patient intake and access services on the first floor, consolidating the medical/surgical ICUs on 2-West, upgrading the surgery suite, converting 3-MOC and 4-MOC for inpatient care, and converting of 5-North, 7-North, and 8-North to office occupancy to allow the demolition of the Cox and Jewett wings. Only the inpatient beds on the third and fourth floors of the older north and west wings would remain, with the balance of the beds located on floors two through six of the newer MOC. A total of $30 million was allocated over the ten-year period for upgrading of the LMH campus.

Recent Utilization Trends at LMH

Lee Memorial Hospital's acute medical/surgical census was reviewed for the previous four years, as shown in Table 9.4. Although admissions had leveled off, length of stay fluctuated, indicating that it too may be leveling off. The resulting average daily census had increased from 152 patients in 1999 to 166 patients in 2002. The average occupancy for 2002 was compared to the peak-month occupancy based on the number of staffed beds. If LMH had only private rooms, an occupancy rate of 90 percent would be a reasonable target to determine the number of beds required based on the peak-month census. Based on a peak-month census of 200 patients, around 222 acute medical/surgical beds would be required during the winter season.

A further review of recent trends in ancillary workload volumes revealed that emergency, CT, and noninvasive cardiology workloads have been growing while surgery and routine imaging workloads remained relatively flat. Nuclear medicine, ultrasound, and endoscopy workloads declined primarily because of a reduction in outpatient volume.

Revised Facility Development Scenarios for LMH

Based on a review of the 1999 facility development strategy for LMH, an evaluation of recent market dynamics and workload trends, and the confirmation of current and future space need, three new scenarios were developed. In all three, it was assumed that the Rehabilitation Hospital would continue to occupy two floors of the MOC and maintain its current license of 60 beds. The complement of medical/surgical beds at LMH would be adjusted over time to reflect the systemwide long-range strategy to decompress the LMH campus and to increase the medical/surgical bed complement at HPMC. The three scenarios identified in 2002 for LMH, summarized in Table 9.5, are as follows.

	1998	1999	2000	2002
Admissions	11,164	12,705	12,410	12,591
Patient days	55,434	61,699	61,837	60,548
Average length of stay	5.0	4.9	5.0	4.8
Average daily census	151.9	169.0	169.4	165.9

Staffed beds	264
Average occupancy	63%

Peak-month census	200
Peak-month occupancy	76%

Scenario 1: Do Nothing. The LMHS board wanted to know what would happen if investment in LMH was limited to only that required to maintain continuous operation over the next ten years, such as the elimination of life safety issues and code noncompliances. In this scenario, infrastructure upgrading would be limited to critical systems such as water, medical vacuum, automatic sprinkler controls, and elevators while the air handling units, emergency generators, and the roof would be replaced. Furnishings and finishes would be upgraded as needed to maintain a clean and professional image. Based on this analysis, it was estimated that $10 million would be required just to maintain LMH over the next decade.

Scenario 2: Maintain the Current Market Share. This scenario included additional investment over the next five years at the LMH campus to prevent market share erosion. In addition to that required in Scenario 1, new projects included the following:

- Upgrading and expanding the surgery suite;

- Consolidating the medical/surgical ICU beds on 2-West adjacent to the surgery suite;

- Demolishing of the older Cox and Jewett wings; and

TABLE 9.5 REVISED FACILITY DEVELOPMENT SCENARIOS FOR LEE MEMORIAL HOSPITAL

	Scenario 1: *Do Nothing*		Scenario 2: *Maintain the Current Market Share*		Scenario 3: *Revitalize the LMH Campus*	
Major actions	Upgrade plant/infrastructure	$ 5.6 M	Consolidate ICUs	$ 4.8 M	Build new clinical building	$ 30.4 M
	Modernize elevators	$ 1.3 M	Expand/upgrade surgery suite	$ 3.0 M	Build new power plant	$ 4.0 M
	Replace roofing	$ 0.5 M	Demolish Cox/Jewett wings	$ 2.0 M	Build new service building	$ 0.8 M
	Upgrade finishes/furnishings	$ 3.0 M	Expand parking/landscaping	$ 0.6 M	Convert 3-MOC to patient care	$ 5.5 M
			+ *Scenario 1 Costs*	*$10.4 M*	Convert 4-MOC to patient care	$ 5.8 M
					Upgrade 4-West	$ 1.0 M
					Demolish north wing/old plant	$ 2.3 M
					+ *Scenario 2 Costs*	*$20.8 M*
New space	None		None		127,000 GSF: Clinical building (100,000 GSF) Service building (15,000 GSF) Power plant (12,000 GSF)	
Space eliminated	None		70,000 GSF (Cox/Jewett wings)		264,000 GSF: North wing/plant (184,000 GSF) Education wing (10,000 GSF) Cox/Jewett (70,000 GSF)	

Space unassigned	15,000+ GSF (7-North/8-North)	26,000+ GSF (7-North/8-North)	None
Bed impact (staffed)	264 Medical/surgical beds 60 Rehab beds 324 Total beds	254 Medical/surgical beds 60 Rehab beds 314 Total beds	200+ Medical/surgical beds 60 Rehab beds 260+ Total beds
Cost	$10.4 M	$20.8 M	$70.6 M

Source: Reprinted with permission from Lee Memorial Health System, Ft. Myers, Florida.

- Improving the main entrance façade, enhancing the landscaping, and expanding patient and visitor parking.

These improvements would cost an additional $10 million to $11 million over the next five years, resulting in a total of $21 million when added to the infrastructure upgrading outlined under Scenario 1.

Scenario 3: Revitalize the LMH Campus. Instead of minimizing investment in LMH, this scenario focuses on revitalizing the LMH campus to enhance its market position and to provide contemporary, albeit resized, facilities. This scenario includes approximately 127,000 BGSF of new construction to replace the older north wing and the Cox and Jewett wings, which would be demolished. In total, approximately 264,000 BGSF would be demolished to make way for the new construction. Key projects would include the following:

- Constructing an inexpensive service building to house materials management, plant engineering, and medical record and film storage currently located in prime space in the MOC; potential replacement of the existing kitchen is also under consideration;

- Constructing a new clinical building to replace the existing ED, imaging center, and surgery suite with the potential for additional inpatient floors;

- Constructing a new energy center (power plant);

- Converting 3-MOC and 4-MOC to inpatient nursing units and upgrading the 4-West nursing unit; and

- Eventually demolishing the north wing.

It was also proposed that selected support services be consolidated at CCH, such as specialty laboratory testing, sterile processing, medical transcription, and information systems. In this scenario, an existing LMHS-owned office building would be retained for administrative offices not requiring a hospital presence.

Selected Facility Development Scenario
Because of LMHS's improving financial position and the renewed development in downtown Ft. Myers and the surrounding area, the

LMHS executive council and board reached consensus on Scenario 3, thus committing to an investment of over $70 million at the LMH campus over the decade.

The building section diagram presented in Figure 9.5 graphically illustrates the revised long-range facility development plan for LMH as described in Scenario 3.

LEE MEMORIAL HEALTH SYSTEM TODAY

The systemwide facility master plan developed in 1999 has continued to guide LMHS's capital investments since its inception, as specific projects are completed and others are transitioned from planning to design and construction. LMHS's executive council was actively involved in translating their vision for the organization into a flexible, long-range capital investment strategy for their multiple campuses. They also recognized the importance of achieving consensus on an overall strategy and related actions before focusing on the bricks and mortar. Because their capital investment strategy provides adequate flexibility, they are able to adjust individual projects over time as market dynamics change.

In early 2005, the Florida Agency for Health Care Administration (ACHA) eliminated their requirement for a Certificate of Need for bed expansion at existing hospitals in high-growth areas. To receive approval for 122 additional beds at the HPMC campus, LMHS had previously made a request to transfer licensed beds from the LMH and CCH campuses to HPMC. LMHS withdrew its Certificate of Need application because it no longer needed to formally transfer licensed beds from one facility to another and could simply add beds where needed without a Certificate of Need. At the same time, the Hospital Corporation of America (HCA) has received approval to construct a new 350-bed hospital in south Lee County (on the site of their existing Gulf Coast Hospital), which could affect LMHS's market share. This new facility is expected to be completed in 2008 and will replace both the existing Gulf Coast Hospital and the Southwest Regional Medical Center.

HealthPark Medical Center

Urgent issues in 1999 concerning medical/surgical and obstetric bed capacity at HPMC were resolved through the creation of several innovative observation and short-stay units (primarily unlicensed beds) as the

FIGURE 9.5 REVISED LONG-RANGE FACILITY DEVELOPMENT PLAN FOR LEE MEMORIAL HOSPITAL

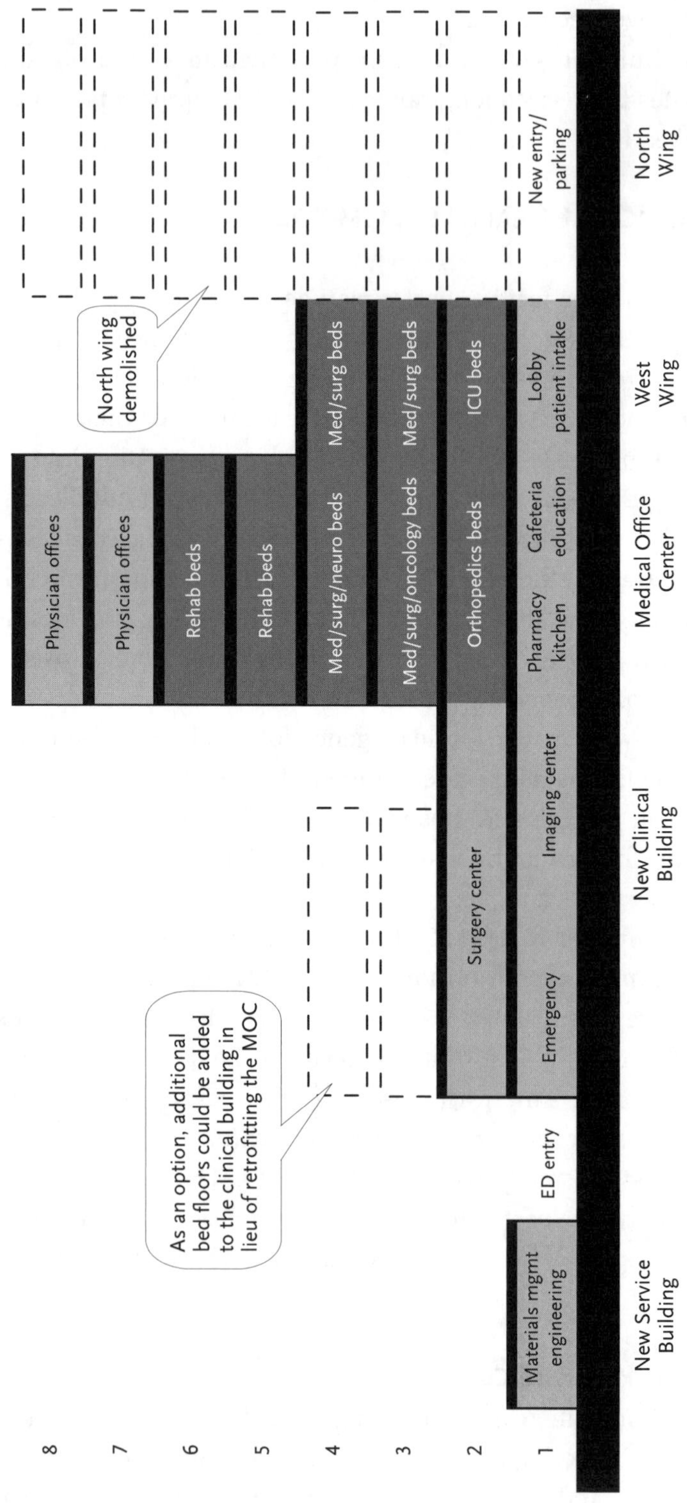

Source: Reprinted with permission from Lee Memorial Health Systems, Ft. Myers, Florida

detailed planning for the construction of new beds commenced. With annual births reaching 3,500, HPMC is no longer using their 36 birthing rooms for single-room maternity care but has created a separate postpartum nursing unit. Groundbreaking occurred in early 2003 for the construction of three additional inpatient floors and a new ancillary building, as well as expansion of the central energy plant. This significant project will increase HPMC's bed complement to 362 beds. Construction is currently ahead of schedule, and completion is expected in late 2005.

Lee Memorial Hospital

The original strategy developed in 1999 to decompress LMH and refocus it as a high-tech facility dedicated to trauma, special surgery (orthopedics, neurosciences, and oncology), rehabilitation, and ambulatory care has remained unchanged today. The updated 2002 facility master plan for LMH proposed a higher level of capital investment at this campus because of LMHS's improving financial position and the renewed development in downtown Ft. Myers. The older Cox and Jewett wings are being demolished as part of the staging for the construction of a new clinical building and the eventual demolition of the north wing.

Cape Coral Hospital

The modest projects originally identified for CCH have been completed, and the consolidation of the clinical laboratory, central sterile, and information systems at CCH are underway. This will provide additional staging space at LMH.

NOTE

1. Lee Memorial Health System granted permisson for this case study.

REFERENCE

Solucient. 2005. *Top 100 Hospitals: National Benchmarks for Success 2004*. Evanston, IL: Solucient, LLC.

CHAPTER TEN

Reconfiguring the First Floor of a Medical Center to Enhance Customer Service and Promote Future Flexibility: A Case Study

T HE CHARLES F. Kettering Memorial Hospital[1] opened in 1964 as a tribute to Charles F. Kettering, the world-renowned American inventor, scientist, and humanitarian. This 522-bed hospital is part of the Kettering Medical Center Network—a not-for-profit regional healthcare system serving the residents of the greater Dayton area and beyond. Charles F. Kettering Memorial Hospital (now known as Kettering Medical Center) is one of the healthcare system's four acute care hospitals.

Kettering Medical Center (KMC) is recognized as a major cardiac center, is noted for its comprehensive cancer program, and has received awards for its stroke, joint replacement, and inpatient rehabilitation programs. The healthcare system has historically strived to provide superb customer service, and in 2004 and 2005, KMC was cited as a Distinguished Hospital for "An Outstanding Patient Experience" by J.D. Power and Associates.

As shown in Figure 10.1, the main facility complex at KMC includes a five-story hospital structure (plus a lower level) with an integrated

FIGURE 10.1 EXISTING FUNCTIONAL LAYOUT OF KETTERING MEDICAL CENTER (BUILDING SECTION DIAGRAM)

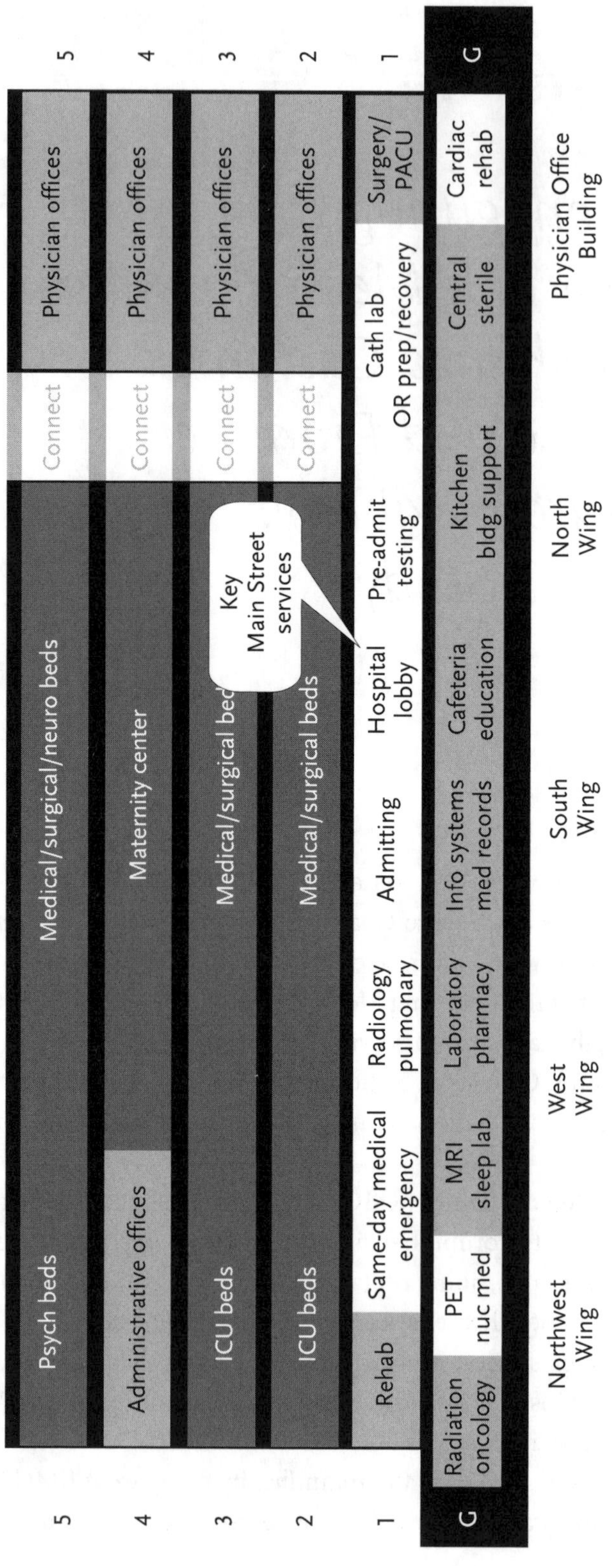

Floor	Northwest Wing	West Wing	South Wing	North Wing		Physician Office Building
5	Psych beds	Medical/surgical/neuro beds			Connect	Physician offices
4	Administrative offices	Maternity center			Connect	Physician offices
3	ICU beds	Medical/surgical beds			Connect	Physician offices
2	ICU beds	Medical/surgical beds			Connect	Physician offices
1	Rehab	Same-day medical emergency	Radiology pulmonary / Admitting	Hospital lobby / Pre-admit testing	Cath lab OR prep/recovery	Surgery/PACU
G	Radiation oncology	PET nuc med / MRI sleep lab	Laboratory pharmacy / Info systems med records	Cafeteria education / Kitchen bldg support	Central sterile	Cardiac rehab

Key: Main Street services

Source: Reprinted with permission from Kettering Medical Center, Kettering, Ohio.

Physician Office Building (POB) that connects to the hospital at each floor level. Diagnostic and treatment services are located primarily on the ground and first floors with inpatient nursing units occupying the upper floors. Floors two through five of the POB are used for physician offices. Building support services such as central sterile processing, kitchen, and materials management are located on the north side of the ground floor along with the cafeteria and education space.

Renovation and upgrading has occurred on the first floor over the past several years based on a concept referred to as the "Main Street" plan. The intent was to implement a staged reconfiguration of the first floor to enhance ambulatory care delivery through convenient access, simplified wayfinding, and coordinated diagnostic and treatment services. Using this approach, KMC leadership can effectively compete with freestanding ambulatory care facilities while avoiding the redundant capital and operational costs often associated with dispersed off-site services. A multiyear facility reconfiguration plan was prepared that includes eight sequential renovation phases. The first two phases of the plan have been completed to date and were focused on a portion of the planned emergency room expansion. Figure 10.2 shows the layout of the first floor at the completion of these first two phases.

KEY COMPONENTS OF THE ORIGINAL PLAN

A primary objective of the original Main Street plan was to create two primary circulation arteries, connecting at the main hospital elevator bank, to simplify patient and visitor circulation. These two circulation arteries are as follows:

1. The north-south corridor, or main street, connects the ED entrance to the south with the main hospital entrance and lobby, surgery reception and check-in area, POB elevators, and POB entrance to the north.

2. The east-west corridor, or side street, connects the main hospital entry and lobby to the east with the reception and check-in areas for the same-day medical services, pulmonary services, endoscopy, radiology, catheterization laboratory, and the northwest entrance and elevators to the west.

FIGURE 10.2 EXISTING FUNCTIONAL LAYOUT OF KETTERING MEDICAL CENTER (FIRST FLOOR)

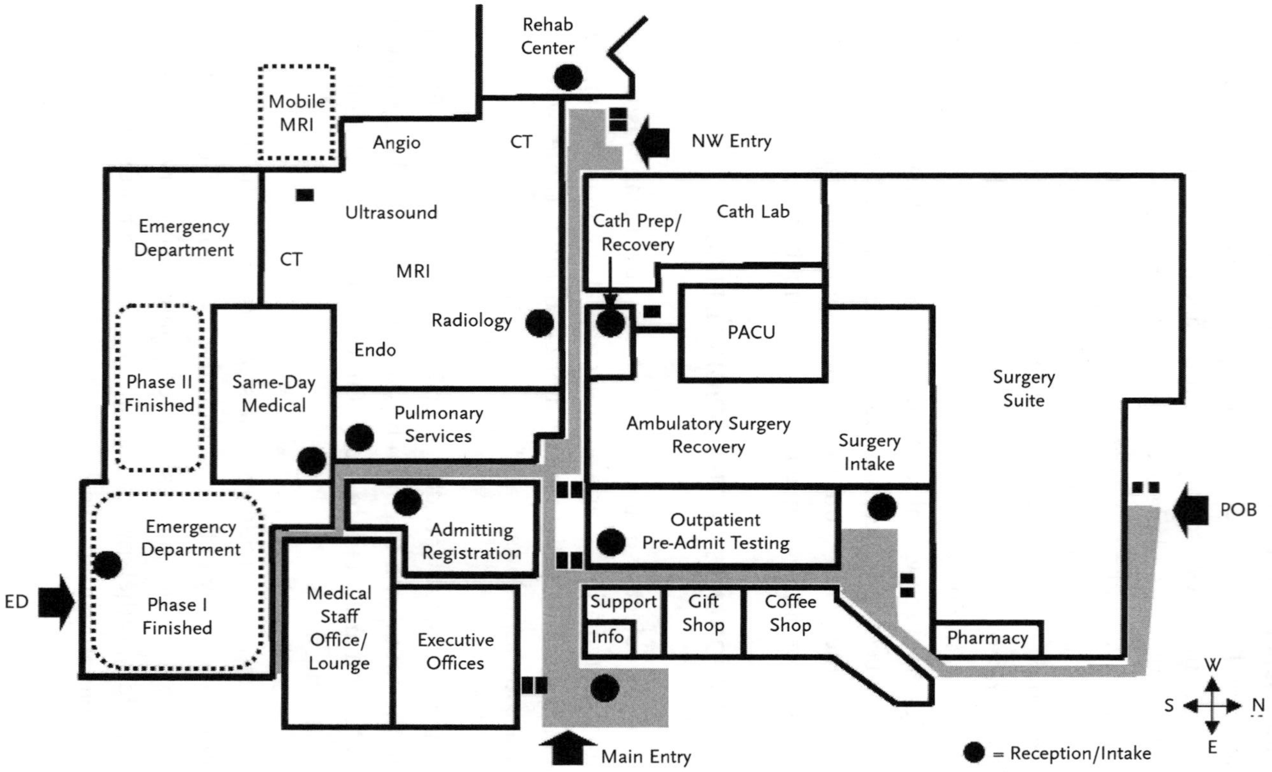

Other key components of this concept include the following:

- The creation of a common reception and check-in area for same-day medical services, pulmonary services, and endoscopy with a contiguous area for inpatient admitting and bed control

- The expansion of same-day medical treatment and recovery space to be shared among multiple departments

- The creation of a new reception and check-in area for medical imaging

- The reconfiguration of medical imaging space to collocate procedure rooms by modality

No significant changes were planned for the services located on the north half of the first floor, including the catheterization laboratory, surgery suite, and outpatient preadmission testing. Also, no changes were envisioned for the existing hospital main lobby and associated customer amenities such as the gift shop, coffee shop, and retail pharmacy. It was assumed that the executive office suite and the recently renovated medical staff office and physician lounge would remain in their current location directly south of the main hospital lobby unless a need to reallocate their space for clinical services was clearly documented.

THE CHALLENGE

In 2004, KMC leadership requested a formal reevaluation of the main street plan. The intent was to solicit an objective assessment of the initial strategy relative to recent workload fluctuations, changes in renovation phasing priorities, and optimal future flexibility. Recommendations to enhance customer wayfinding—for example, site access, signage, external entrances, and internal destinations—were also solicited for incorporation into the revised first-floor reconfiguration plan.

Related planning initiatives were also underway and needed to be integrated with the first-floor reconfiguration strategy as follows:

- Specific studies were underway to assess and improve surgery operations and to develop a systemwide strategic plan for cardiovascular services.

- An interdisciplinary task force was developing a common systemwide strategy and objectives for admitting and outpatient registration.

- Preliminary planning to increase the number of private patient rooms was in process.

Specific questions to be addressed as part of this new planning effort included the following:

- Should the ongoing reconfiguration of the ground and first floor levels continue to follow the Main Street plan developed several years ago? Are the workload and corresponding space projections still valid?

- How should preadmission testing ideally be organized? How can patient intake and access services be reconfigured to enhance customer service, to increase staffing efficiency, and to optimize space utilization?

- How can upgrading of the radiology department be expedited? Should MRI ultimately be consolidated on the ground floor, directly below the radiology department? Should pulmonary rehabilitation be relocated to the ground floor contiguous with cardiac rehabilitation? What is the appropriate role, staffing, and space for the same-day medical service?

- What is the current capacity of major diagnostic and treatment services based on the current number of procedure rooms, equipment, and support space? Could operational changes or equipment upgrading increase capacity in lieu of facility expansion?

- Which departments are currently experiencing the greatest space deficiencies? Are there other facility deficiencies that do not necessary involve more space, such as an inadequate functional layout and internal configuration; inappropriate location; and other operational, equipment, or technology issues? What amount of growth is anticipated for each service within the next five years? What additional space will be required?

- What is the "highest and best use" of services to be located on the first floor? Ground floor?

- How can facility reconfiguration and improved signage facilitate customer wayfinding on the ground and first floors?

THE PLANNING PROCESS

The process for reconfiguration of the first floor of KMC included the following activities:

- A review of the original main street plan and the evolving concerns about the remaining implementation phases

- An assessment of the major services located on the first floor relative to their current situation, recent utilization trends, current and future space need, and outstanding issues

- The development of a revised first-floor reconfiguration plan based on key strategies and related actions

A steering committee was established that was led by the senior executive officer for administration and included the vice presidents for clinical services and nursing. Work sessions also included the director of facility management and KMC's architect of record. Periodic progress reports were made to the KMC executive council to review preliminary conclusions and recommendations.

After review of the original main street plan, representatives from KMC's senior leadership team were interviewed to identify their evolving concerns about the remaining implementation phases. At the same time, baseline data were collected for the major services "in play" using a facility planning questionnaire. Upon receiving and reviewing the questionnaires, interviews were also conducted with selected department and service-line managers. Recent workload trends were analyzed and compared to current resource utilization such as staff, equipment, and space. Current and future space need was determined based on future workload forecasts, proposed operational changes, and new technology investments rather than solely on department managers' perceptions. The space projections and priorities were then translated into a revised first-floor reconfiguration strategy, and corresponding actions were reviewed with the steering committee prior to finalization.

EVOLVING CONCERNS ABOUT THE REMAINING
IMPLEMENTATION PHASES

At this critical juncture, with the first two phases of construction completed, KMC leadership had several concerns about the continued implementation of the original plan. A key concern was that the various departments on the first floor were being planned in silos with inadequate cooperation and coordination among department management and staff to ensure the optimal sharing of resources and future flexibility. At the same time, new leadership wanted to challenge the status quo. Specific concerns are discussed below.

Expansion of the Catheterization Laboratory Was Not Addressed

Invasive cardiology procedures were growing, particularly electrophysiology (EP) and implant procedures, which are more time consuming than traditional diagnostic catheterizations. There are currently four procedure rooms (with one dedicated for EP), an adjacent seven-bay preparation and recovery area, and limited support space. The capacity of the current facilities is severely constrained by the age of the equipment and the lack of preparation, holding, and recovery space. Limited space on the first floor for outpatient preparation and recovery (almost half of the current cath volume) creates a labor-intensive process of admitting patients at the outpatient preadmission testing (OPAT) area, transferring them to a third-floor nursing unit for preparation and holding, bringing them down to the first-floor catheterization laboratory for their procedure, and then transferring them back up to the third floor for recovery and subsequent discharge. Families are encouraged to wait in the surgical waiting area at the north end of the first floor. A total of 6,900 DGSF is provided, which is minimal for a four-procedure room catheterization laboratory.

Static Surgery Volume and Surplus Capacity

As a result of the healthcare system's success in developing freestanding outpatient surgery facilities in partnership with their surgeons, outpatient surgery at KMC had leveled off from 2001 to 2003. At the same time, inpatient surgery had been relatively static with the proliferation of minimally invasive procedures and the shift to same-day procedures.

In 2003, outpatients represented 56 percent of the total surgical patients. With an average of 37 outpatients per day and 30 outpatient preparation and recovery bays, surplus capacity is available, particularly with the trend toward shorter recovery times with shorter-acting anesthetics. On two days per week, the surgery department does not use two of the eight outpatient recovery pods, which is notable because one of these pods abuts the existing catheterization preparation and recovery space. The 20 ORs and cysto room also appear to have ample capacity based on standard benchmarks (800 annual cases per OR at KMC versus a benchmark of 950–1,000). Although several scenarios were developed to anticipate OR need over the next five years, it appears that there would be sufficient ORs to accommodate even the most aggressive scenario if room turnover were improved or hours of operation extended.

Reconfiguration of Medical Imaging Was Not a High Priority

In the original main street plan, reconfiguration of imaging services does not occur until the final phase of renovation. The imaging rooms are currently fragmented with modalities split—for example, CT and MRI—and outpatient reception, intake, and waiting space is limited. Most of the radiographic and fluoroscopic rooms and both angiography rooms need to be upgraded, and ultrasound is congested with minimal patient privacy. Inadequate CT and ultrasound capacity is becoming a concern with steadily increasing volumes.

A single MRI room is located within the department, which is supplemented by a temporary mobile unit that will eventually be replaced. At the same time, the original MRI procedure room still exists directly below on the ground floor in space that has been essentially "mothballed." Nuclear medicine and PET are also located directly below on the ground floor along with noninvasive cardiology and radiation oncology. Recent changes include the installation of a new high-speed CT within the radiation oncology area, which could be used for inpatients. Also, the development of a full-service breast-imaging center in the POB will eliminate the need for mammography rooms within the hospital.

In the original main street plan, a central reception and intake area was planned for imaging services, and the two CT rooms will be collocated. However, no reconfiguration of MRI or ultrasound is planned. The need to replace the angiography equipment and the underutilized x-ray room on the third floor of the POB, which averages 300 procedures per month, were also not addressed in the original plan.

Potential Surplus ED Capacity

With 41 ED treatment bays planned for 39,000 annual visits, the concerns were that the ED was being overplanned, particularly because the potential sharing of space between same-day medical services and the ED was not addressed. Emergency department volumes were relatively flat from 2001 through 2003 because of KMC's efforts to provide cost-effective alternate settings for care delivery. The five-year projection of ED treatment bays indicated that 41 treatment bays would be sufficient space to accommodate even the most aggressive scenario with no improvement in treatment room turnaround time.

Overplanned Same-Day Medical Treatment Bays

Same-day medical services currently uses 16 bays and six chairs to accommodate a variety of medical procedures and also recovers all outpatients receiving conscious sedation, such as endoscopy and medical imaging. Two procedure rooms are dedicated for endoscopy, and the pulmonary services department uses various testing and treatment spaces along with an exercise room. All of these services experience a severe shortage of support space such as patient intake, storage, and staff work areas.

The same-day medical workload has been stable over the past three years. The average visit was 106 minutes in 2003, and approximately 37 percent of the procedures averaged less than one hour. Pulmonary diagnostic and respiratory care procedures have also been stable with the majority of procedures performed on inpatients.

On the other hand, pulmonary rehabilitation visits have increased significantly, with outpatients representing 65 percent of the workload. Endoscopy procedures have increased slightly with outpatients currently representing 58 percent of the total volume.

A total of 36 shared preparation and recovery bays are planned for the new same-day medical unit that will occupy 17,000 DGSF in the middle of the first floor. With a projected average of 56 visits per day and an average turnover time of less than two hours, 36 bays will provide more than ample capacity.

Outpatient Preadmission Testing (OPAT) and Patient Access Services Are Being Reevaluated

No changes to the existing OPAT area were planned in the original main street plan. The current organization of services and physical configuration is extremely confusing for customers, including the signage, destinations, and processes. The space is ample but inappropriately allocated and configured as follows:

- The admitting and registration area is remote from the main lobby, reception desk, and other related services; customers often inadvertently wait in the OPAT area regardless of their correct destination, such as admitting and registration or surgery check-in.

- There is a surplus of admitting cubicles and exam rooms with the transition to preregistration and phone interviewing.

- One-third of the existing OPAT space was formerly an imaging suite with four exam rooms and is not currenlty used.

Several operational changes are underway systemwide that will affect the need for central patient access and OPAT space on the first floor. These include the reevaluation of face-to-face presurgery and preadmission screening, the decentralization of registrars such as in the imaging and surgery waiting areas, the upgrading of the health system's web site to include a patient portal, and the implementation of barcoding for patient tracking. Currently, there are six to seven clerks who primarily contact patients by phone and do not require a location on the first floor. As a future systemwide vision for patient admission and registration evolves, staff involved in face-to-face contact will be even less needed.

The Hospital Main Entry and Signage Were Not Addressed

The "ceremonial" main entrance is not well utilized and only includes a small reception and information desk staffed by volunteers rather than a formal customer service function. Alternately, the surgery waiting area down the hallway is frequently congested. Signage is inconsistent, contains too much information (which impedes decision making), and is not reinforced in the parking garage and at building entry points.

DEVELOPMENT OF KEY STRATEGIES AND ACTIONS

Five strategies were developed to guide reconfiguration of the first floor, and specific actions were identified for each strategy:

- Strategy 1: Improve customer wayfinding, convenience, and amenities

- Strategy 2: Reconfigure medical imaging to provide state-of-the-art technology, enhance patient flow, and improve staff efficiency

- Strategy 3: Provide flexible, state-of-the-art interventional procedure rooms and support space

- Strategy 4: Reconfigure medical procedure and recovery space to enhance patient flow and improve staff efficiency

- Strategy 5: Rethink the OPAT area as express services

The revised reconfiguration plan and wayfinding concept for the first floor is presented in Figure 10.3.

Strategy 1: Improve Customer Wayfinding, Convenience, and Amenities

This strategy includes seven major actions:

1. Consistent with the original main street plan, use the ED, main entrance, POB, and northwest lobbies as prominent wayfinding "nodes" or destinations, reinforcing the primary north-south corridor and the secondary east-west corridor.

2. Create a single customer service center at the intersection of the north-south and east-west corridors, directly accessible from the main hospital lobby and serving as a hub from which to coordinate the following customer services, patient processing functions, and amenities:

   - Reception, information, and wayfinding

   - Admitting and outpatient registration

   - Financial counseling, insurance verification, and cashiering

   - Family and visitor lounge

   - Other amenities such as a gift shop, coffee cart, etc.

3. Staff the customer service center reception desk with professional, cross-trained facilitators familiar with information, registration,

Figure 10.3 Proposed Floor Layout for Kettering Medical Center (First Floor)

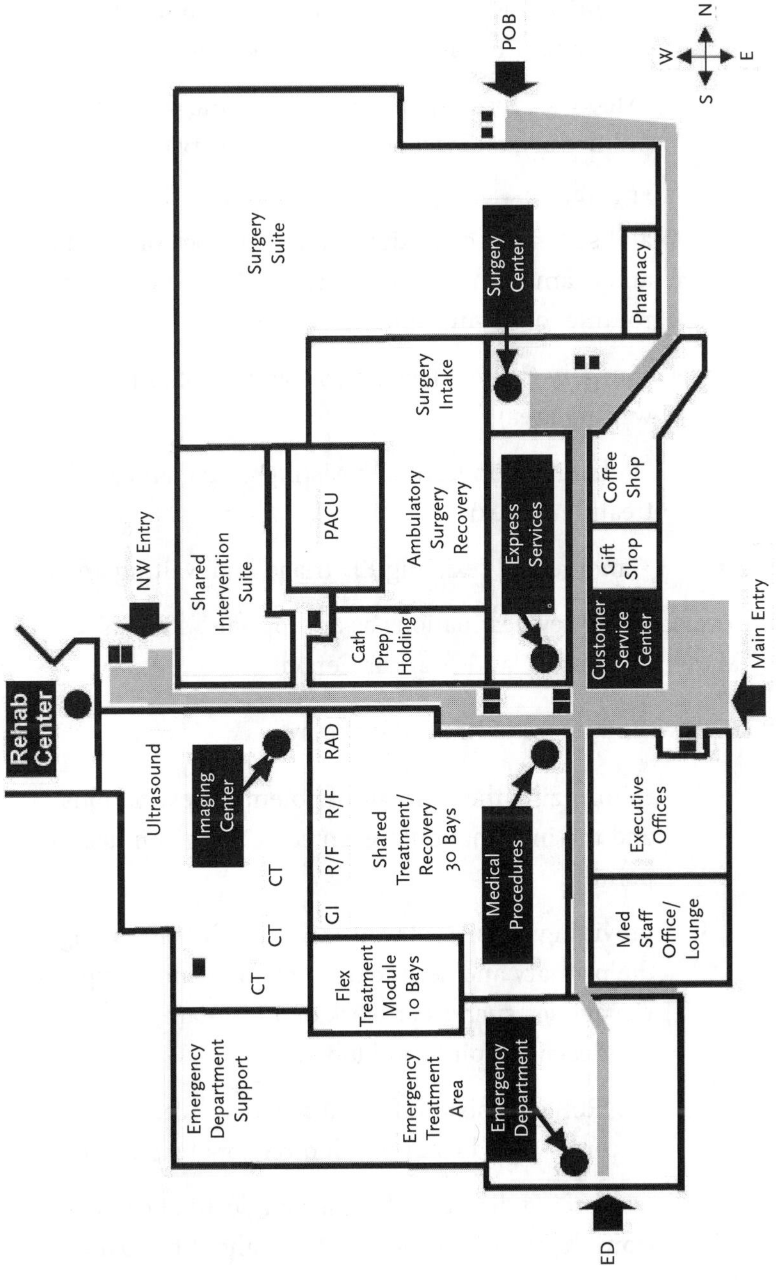

and scheduling similar to a hotel reception desk; use electronic kiosks and better signage to facilitate wayfinding.

4. Create a limited number of customer reception and check-in destinations for services on the first floor to facilitate wayfinding and enhance operational efficiency, including the following:

- "Imaging Center," including radiology; ultrasound; CT; MRI; and optionally, check-in for nuclear medicine, PET, and noninvasive cardiology

- "Medical Procedures," including same-day medical, pulmonary, endoscopy, and related services

- "Express Services," including phlebotomy and specimen collection, multipurpose consultation and exam rooms, simple x-rays, EKGs, and other routine, quick-turnaround services

- "Surgery Center" (existing surgery check-in and waiting area)

- "Rehabilitation Center" (existing intake and treatment area)

- "Emergency" (existing ED triage and waiting area)

5. Develop other key destinations as appropriate, such as the "POB," "Maternity Center," and "Cancer Center."

6. Improve and upgrade KMC signage by

- minimizing the number of potential destinations and the information presented at any given decision point;

- providing consistent wall and floor finishes along the primary and secondary corridors, and using visual cues such as artwork or a fountain to identify key decision points and lobbies;

- providing consistent format and typeface, placement, and color for all directional signs; and

- reinforcing directional signs and destination names from the initial site access, throughout the parking garage, at building entrance points, and continuing to the point of service.

7. Reinforce signage at the ground floor for outpatient services and amenities to be maintained on this floor level, particularly at the main and northwest elevators.

Strategy 2: Reconfigure Medical Imaging to Provide State-of-the-Art Technology, Enhance Patient Flow, and Improve Staff Efficiency

This strategy includes three major actions:

1. Create a central reception and check-in area (imaging center) easily accessible from the primary and secondary circulation corridors.

2. Collocate similar modalities to facilitate efficient staffing—for example, radiographic and fluoroscopic, CT, and MRI—and do the following:

   • Proceed with the original plan to collocate routine x-ray, R/F, endoscopy, and bronchoscopy procedure rooms.

   • Collocate the two CT rooms, and provide space for a potential third CT room.

   • Create a pod of two to three MRI rooms on the ground floor in unassigned space, and discontinue use of the mobile unit.

3. Equip all procedures rooms with state-of-the-art digital equipment.

Strategy 3: Provide Flexible, State-of-the-Art Interventional Procedure Rooms and Support Space

This strategy includes four major actions:

1. Upgrade invasive cardiology equipment and procedure rooms.

2. Upgrade angiography rooms and support space.

3. Collocate all interventional procedure rooms to provide optimal future flexibility such as the following:

- Cardiac catheterization and EP

- Angiography and interventional radiology

- Surgical operating rooms

4. Create a dedicated patient preparation and recovery area for invasive cardiology (using a portion of the existing ambulatory surgery recovery space) where outpatient catheterizations can be checked-in, prepared, and recovered on the first floor; utilize the same-day medical recovery space as needed for overflow.

Strategy 4: Reconfigure Medical Procedure and Recovery Space to Enhance Patient Flow and Improve Staff Efficiency

This strategy includes four major actions:

1. Create a central reception and check-in area (medical procedures) for same-day medical, endoscopy, pulmonary, and other related services that are easily accessible from the primary and secondary circulation corridors.

2. Proceed with the plan to collocate the gastrointestinal (GI) and pulmonary procedure rooms with R/F imaging rooms.

3. Relocate pulmonary rehabilitation to the ground floor contiguous with cardiac rehabilitation, and utilize its dedicated entrance and parking area.

4. Create a flexible ten-bay treatment bay module that can be used by both ED and same-day medical patients depending on demand—for example, by shift, seasonally, or over time as workloads fluctuate.

Strategy 5: Rethink the OPAT Area as Express Services

This strategy includes five major actions:

1. Maintain the existing OPAT entrance, phlebotomy and specimen collection area, and classroom.

2. Discontinue use of OPAT space for the pain clinic, which should be incorporated into the same-day medical space.

3. Reactivate the existing x-ray room, and close the x-ray and phlebotomy and specimen collection satellite on the third floor of the POB.

4. Maintain two to three exam rooms for preadmission and presurgery testing and consultations, assuming face-to-face interaction will be minimized.

5. Utilize the balance of the existing OPAT space for other related routine, quick-turnaround services.

KETTERING MEDICAL CENTER TODAY

The proposed first-floor reconfiguration strategies and actions were approved by the KMC executive council. The healthcare system's architect of record is developing revised architectural plans for the first and ground floors along with an updated phasing/implementation schedule. A signage study was also conducted to identify interim signage changes that could be made immediately to improve patient and visitor wayfinding prior to completion of the entire renovation plan. Other proposed changes are also being expedited, such as creation of the customer service center and the flexible reassignment of ambulatory surgery recovery bays as needed by other services such as cardiac catheterization. Part of the success of the revised planning process can be attributed to new managers in the ED, surgery suite, and outpatient preadmission testing department who are focused on the needs of KMC's patients rather than on maintaining their own individual turfs.

NOTE

1. Kettering Medical Center granted permission for this case study.

CHAPTER ELEVEN

Optimizing Current and Future Flexibility

T HE TERM *FLEXIBILITY* has become somewhat overused today. It is repeated as a mantra among healthcare planners and design architects. By definition, it means "adaptable" or "adjustable to change." In reality, achieving flexibility often requires that physicians, department managers, and staff relinquish absolute control over their space and equipment for the greater good of the organization.

WHY IS FLEXIBILITY IMPORTANT?

Many of the reasons why we need to provide flexible and adaptable healthcare facilities have already been addressed in previous chapters of this book. Some of these reasons include the following:

- The unpredictable healthcare environment with fluctuating demand driven by changing reimbursement, new regulations, and media attention;

- The blending and melding of many diagnostic and treatment modalities with advances in technology;

- Staffing shortages in many specialties that necessitate the cross-training of staff and the creation of new job descriptions;

- Electronic information management that eliminates the need for physical proximity; and

- Limited access to capital that requires ever more efficient utilization of all resources, including staff, equipment, and space.

DIFFERENT WAYS OF ACHIEVING FLEXIBILITY

Facilities should be planned to *optimize current utilization* as well as to *provide flexible space that can be adapted over time*. Some ways to achieve flexibility include the following:

Planning Multiuse or Shared Facility Components

This enables a healthcare organization to use their space efficiently and to balance workload peaks and valleys. Examples of multiuse spaces include the following:

- Acuity adaptable, or "universal," patient rooms can be adapted for most levels of acuity by altering staffing levels and equipment. This concept can reduce costly patient transfers during an increasingly short length of stay, provide improved continuity of care, and reduce medical errors.

- Time-share clinic space can be leased by physicians—for example, patient reception and intake areas, exam rooms, offices, and support space—by the day of week as needed, thus reducing fixed costs.

- Multiuse procedure rooms can accommodate various procedures as needed using different types of portable equipment such as EKG and ultrasound.

- Alternate space use by shift, such as by using an adjacent occupational medicine clinic or same-day medical procedure unit for treating ED fast-track patients during the evening or night shift, or by holding ED patients in the surgery suite recovery area during the evening for observation or while waiting for an inpatient bed to become available.

- Collocation of selected procedure rooms so that they can share the same patient reception and intake, preparation, recovery, and support space—for example, the collocation of various imaging modalities, invasive cardiology and angiography, or endoscopy and surgery.

Planning Flexible Space That Can Be Adapted Over Time

This will accommodate shifts in program focus and fluctuating utilization and can reduce long-term renovation costs. This includes space that can be easily adapted for a different functional use over time by replacing the equipment, adding a second bed, or reassigning offices and workstations to another department. In addition to the acuity adaptable patient rooms mentioned above, other examples of adaptable spaces include the following:

- Flexible diagnostic and treatment center with a central patient reception and intake area, preparation and recovery area, shared staff facilities, and a mix of large and small procedure rooms where equipment can be changed and upgraded over time. This is in contrast to the traditional approach of planning dispersed and fragmented departments such as radiology, CT, nuclear medicine, cardiology, and ultrasound.

- Flexible customer service space using a one-stop shopping concept to accommodate admitting and registration, financial counseling, cashiering, scheduling, and other similar services that require face-to-face customer interaction. With flexible offices and cubicles (and cross-trained staff), services can be adapted to the customers' needs over time.

- Generic administrative office suites to be used by various administrative and support staff who do not require face-to-face customer contact. Space can be reassigned over time in response to organizational changes, thus eliminating department turf issues and improving overall space utilization.

Unbundling Selected Services

Rather than embedding everything into the hospital structure, this strategy not only can reduce an organization's initial capital investment but also can facilitate future space reallocation, contraction, and expansion as workloads, staffing, and operational processes change over time. Some examples include the following:

- Relocation of routine, high-volume outpatient services in separate facilities (on or off campus) with dedicated parking and convenient access—for example, primary care clinics; selected high-volume outpatient services; or recurring or chronic outpatient services such as rehabilitation, chemotherapy, and dialysis.

- Consolidation of building support services into a separate service building—for example, supply, processing, and distribution functions—using space that is less expensive to construct and renovate over time as operational systems, technology, and work processes change.

- Relocation of administrative offices for staff who are not involved in direct patient care outside the hospital (on site or off site) in less expensive and adaptable office building space.

Leasing Space

This strategy, versus buying or building, when appropriate allows an organization to limit its capital investment and long-term risk. This may include leasing space off site for administrative offices and new or expanding outpatient programs. Some healthcare organizations may choose to lease space such as a hotel conference room or a school auditorium for periodic in-service or community education in lieu of constructing an education center on the hospital campus. Interior systems furniture and other building elements may also be leased by making an arrangement with a manufacturer to take stewardship over the product's life, including putting it together, refreshing it, and recycling it for a reasonable fee. Some healthcare organizations also keep up with changes in technology by leasing imaging equipment or by paying based on its use rather than buying the equipment outright (Sandrick 2005).

Building a Flexible Infrastructure

Done with long-span joists and interstitial space (although not generally addressed in predesign planning), this provides a cost-effective way to adapt to ongoing changes over the life of a building. When you embed everything in the building so the pipes and wires are inside the walls, floors, and ceiling, it is almost impossible to reconfigure any space without major construction. If you build your hospital more like a shopping center, with a huge superstructure and interiors that can come and go at will, you will have an adaptable tool for delivering healthcare (Sandrick 2005).

DEVELOPING SPACE STANDARDS AND PLANNING GENERIC SPACES

Future flexibility can also be achieved by developing generic space standards for rooms that accommodate similar functions. Cost savings will ultimately occur as these rooms are similarly sized and finished instead of tailored to individual occupants, even though the actual equipment may vary over time. Examples of generic spaces include the following:

- Private patient rooms (acuity-adaptable)

- Small procedure rooms (ultrasound and EKG)

- Large imaging and procedure rooms (CT, PET, and nuclear medicine)

- Interventional and surgical procedure rooms (catheterization, EP, angiography, peripheral vascular, and invasive and minimally invasive surgery)

- Medical procedure cubicles (transfusions, chemotherapy, liver biopsies, recovery from conscious sedation, and fast-track emergency treatment)

- Administrative workstations, cubicles, private offices, and conference rooms

REDESIGNING THE HEALTHCARE CAMPUS

Redesigning the healthcare campus around similar functions and categories of space can facilitate short-term and long-range flexibility. However, strict adherence to the traditional department boundaries may need to be sacrificed. Potential buildings or functional components for the flexible healthcare campus of the future may include the following:

- Patient care units for overnight and multiple-day stays, day recovery centers, and shared diagnostic and treatment services (inpatient and outpatient) in a structure built to traditional hospital building codes

- One or more adjoining medical office buildings (built as outpatient facilities) for physician specialists and related outpatient services

- Specialty centers of excellence to provide one-stop shopping for target service lines, such as cardiology and cancer care, with collocated diagnostic, treatment, and support services

- Separate facilities (on or off campus) with dedicated parking for primary care; selected high-volume outpatient services and recurring and chronic outpatient care such as physical therapy, dialysis, and behavioral health

- A separate service center for supply, processing, and distribution functions

- An administrative office building for administrative and support staff who are not involved in direct patient care or face-to-face customer contact

Other freestanding components could also include long-term care and assisted-living facilities, an education center, fitness/wellness center, and a daycare facility for the children or elderly dependents of employees. Complementary medicine and retail services may also be provided, combined with or adjacent to high-volume traffic areas such as the main entrance or the medical office building.

REFERENCE

Sandrick, K. 2005. "Flextime: Hospital Spaces Bend to Meet Changing Demand." *Health Facilities Management* (18) 3.

CHAPTER TWELVE

Ensuring Success: Optimizing Your Capital Investments

"Long-range planning does not deal with future decisions, but with the future of present decisions."

—Peter F. Drucker (1974)

WHETHER YOU ARE embarking on a major hospital replacement project, reconfiguring your current facilities, or simply upgrading a specific department or service line, the following summary guidelines should help you optimize your capital investments in facilities and increase your likelihood of success.

DEPLOY A FORMAL PREDESIGN PLANNING PROCESS

The primary purpose of this book is to communicate the importance of the predesign planning process. Decisions made during this stage of facility planning have the greatest impact on long-term operational costs and future flexibility, in addition to the initial cost of the bricks and mortar. Whether you use a top-down or a bottom-up approach, integrating facility planning with your strategic (market) analysis, operations improvement, and technology planning efforts will allow you to make decisions with confidence and to move quickly into implementation.

RETHINK CURRENT ORGANIZATIONAL AND OPERATIONAL MODELS AND USE OF TECHNOLOGY

The investment of significant dollars in new or renovated facilities is a rare opportunity for an organization to rethink its current patient care delivery model, operational systems and processes, and use of technology. Department managers should be encouraged to visualize delivering patient care beyond their individual silos. Cross-departmental task forces should be assembled to focus on common patient needs and operational processes to enhance customer satisfaction, provide efficient resource utilization, and promote future flexibility.

SEPARATE PERCEPTION FROM REALITY

Because many factors affect the patient's and staff's perception of inadequate facilities, understanding the actual facility issues before investing millions of dollars in renovation or new construction is important. A foundation of data and rigorous analyses should support the wish lists of department managers and physicians. At the same time, the relationship of the initial first impression to customer satisfaction should not be overemphasized.

DEVELOP REALISTIC RETURN-ON-INVESTMENT ASSUMPTIONS

In the past, many healthcare organizations employed the "build it and they will come" approach to facility planning. Although some organizations were successful, others were faced with underutilized facilities and increased operational costs as revenues remained flat. An investment of dollars in healthcare facilities should be based on a sound business plan that forecasts future revenue and anticipates future operational costs.

USE INDUSTRY BENCHMARKS, RULES OF THUMB, AND BEST PRACTICES FOR VALIDATION

The use of industry benchmarks and rules of thumb, along with a review of best practices around the country and internationally, provides external validation of your plans and may introduce your organization to new concepts and opportunities. This is particularly important when a bottom-up planning process is employed or when department managers have a long tenure with a single organization. Alternately, when a top-down approach is used, the leadership's vision must be communicated to the staff who will eventually occupy the new facilities. Site visits to other healthcare facilities and conversations with department managers and physicians who have implemented innovative operational concepts and technologies can save untold future operational and capital dollars.

FOCUS ON THE CUSTOMER

Although providing superb patient care is always the focus of a healthcare organization's mission, patients are not the only customers. Physicians, employees, employers, payers, and family members and visitors all have unique needs that must be considered during the facility planning process.

OPTIMIZE CURRENT AND FUTURE FLEXIBILITY

As described in Chapter 11, there are a number of ways to optimize current and future flexibility that can reduce short-term capital and operational costs as well as minimize long-term renovation costs.

REFERENCE

Drucker, P. 1974. *Management: Tasks, Responsibilities, Practices.* New York: Harper & Row.

About the Author

Cynthia Hayward, AIA, FAAHC, is principal and founder of Hayward & Associates, LLC in Ann Arbor, Michigan, a national consulting firm specializing in predesign planning for healthcare facilities. She has assisted hundreds of diverse healthcare organizations over the past 25 years to economically and efficiently plan their capital investments. For 20 years, she was a partner with a healthcare management consulting firm (Chi Systems, Inc., which became The Chi Group) until she founded Hayward & Associates. Her unique approach integrates facility planning with market demand analysis and service-line planning, operations improvement, and investments in new equipment and information technology.

In addition to her consulting activities, Ms. Hayward has had a long history in research and development relative to healthcare facility planning. In the mid-1970s, she was part of a team contracted by the U.S. Department of Health and Human Services to develop a generic healthcare facility planning process for hospitals across the United States. In the early 1980s, she served as project director for a five-year contract with National Health and Welfare Canada to develop a series (Evaluation and Space Programming Methodology Series) of space planning methodologies for healthcare facilities. In addition to their widespread utilization in Canada, these methodologies were widely used by regulatory agencies, architects, and hospital planners throughout the United States for the subsequent decade. Ms. Hayward is also the author of *SpaceMed™—A Space Planning Guide for Healthcare Facilities* (see www.space-med.com), which includes a step-by-step workbook and a CD with detailed space planning templates.

Ms. Hayward has been a speaker at regional, national, and international conferences on issues relating to predesign planning and capital investment, including conferences sponsored by the American College of Healthcare Executives, Healthcare Financial Management Association, American Hospital Association, and the American Institute of Architects.

Ms. Hayward has a master of architecture degree from the University of Michigan and is a licensed architect (Michigan). She is also a Fellow of the American Association of Healthcare Consultants and a founding member of the American College of Healthcare Architects.